Mental and Emotional Through Yoga

CU00468412

Mental and Emotional Healing Through Yoga combines key research on the intersection of yoga and mental health with a client-centered, step-by-step framework that can be applied to a range of complex mental and emotional disorders. The book guides readers through the initial intake of the first client session and the development of subsequent sessions, providing case examples from the author's practice to show how yoga's mind–body connection facilitates recuperation and healing. While well-grounded in research and case studies, the book is also highly readable, making it accessible to professionals such as psychotherapists and yoga therapists, as well as individuals and families struggling with mental health issues.

Ghada Osman, PhD, LMFT, C-IAYT, E-RYT 500, is a psychotherapist, certified yoga therapist, yoga teacher, and AFAA-certified aerobics instructor. In her private practice, she specializes in helping clients cope with mental health issues using non-traditional therapies, especially yoga. Before entering private practice, she was professor and chair at San Diego State University.

Mental and Emotional Healing Through Yoga

A Guiding Framework for Therapists and Their Clients

Ghada Osman
Photographs by Cameron Gary

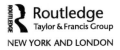
Routledge
Taylor & Francis Group

NEW YORK AND LONDON

First published 2019
by Routledge
711 Third Avenue, New York, NY 10017

and by Routledge
2 Park Square, Milton Park, Abingdon, Oxon, OX14 4RN

Routledge is an imprint of the Taylor & Francis Group, an informa business

Library of Congress Cataloging-in-Publication Data
A catalog record for this title has been requested

ISBN: 978-1-138-04499-9 (hbk)
ISBN: 978-1-138-04500-2 (pbk)
ISBN: 978-1-315-16424-3 (ebk)

Typeset in Garamond
by Out of House Publishing

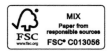

Printed and bound in Great Britain by
TJ International Ltd, Padstow, Cornwall

In gratitude for all that the path of yoga has offered me ...

Contents

Acknowledgments

The completion of this book is not only the culmination of a writing journey, but also a point on a yoga path that began in 1997 at a Total Woman gym in Glendale, California, when I left my first class knowing that somehow, something within me was different after the experience. For their invaluable support on the writing journey, I would like to thank my editor Anna Moore for her enthusiasm about the project from the very start and the seamless way in which she shepherded it, Nina Guttapalle for her efficient and creative assistance with various key aspects of this book, Céline Durassier for her impeccable management of this project, and Sue Clements for her meticulous attention to detail and remarkable copyediting. For their guidance on the yoga path, I would like to thank all my yoga instructors in the past 20+ years, especially the teachers who guided my 500-hour training at the Kripalu Center for Yoga & Health in Lenox, Massachusetts.

The seeds of training students on the use of yoga for mental health began with a conversation over a decade ago with my good friend Melinda Atkins, now director of AUM hOMe Shala, at the time of the first International Association of Yoga Therapists (IAYT) conference in Los Angeles in January 2007. I am immensely grateful to Melinda for her vision, as well as for her continued enthusiasm and hard work that has led to our current programs: 40-hour and 100-hour certifications in yoga for mental health. I would like to thank the scores of students whom I have taught in Florida and California, both the yoga therapists embracing work with emotional health and the psychotherapists embracing work with yoga.

The support of countless people in my life facilitated my work on this project. For their friendship, and therefore for making me a happier person as I was writing, I would like to thank especially Claudia Angelelli and Christian Degueldre, Michael Borgstrom, Elizabeth Colwill, Ann and Ken Gary, Peri Good and Jeff Kaplan, Nina Ronstadt, Elizabeth Sacca, Kristen Stilt, Latha Varadarajan, and Eve Yoshi. A special debt goes to my remarkably gifted therapist friends Jim Reiser, Annie Robershaw, and Rosalind Solo, who have helped me to be not only a happier person but also a better therapist. The greatest debt there goes to my friend and mentor Donald Hanley (he is the mentor mentioned in Chapters 2 and 5), who taught me so much, most significantly how to be a therapist who is also an actual human being. A special thanks to those who graciously and good-naturedly modeled for this book: Farid Abdel-Nour, Camille Forbes, Cameron Gary, and Eve Yoshi.

There are three people in particular whom I would like to thank. The first is Farid Abdel-Nour, for his nurturing, close friendship throughout the decades and his invaluable questions and prompts as I ironed out the first portion of this book in my mind. The second is my sister-friend Camille Forbes, for her enthusiasm about the project from its inception, her reading of and feedback on portions of this book despite her being inundated with other obligations, and her wholehearted encouragement of everything I do. Finally, my husband Cameron Gary, who supported me in every conceivable way throughout this project, serving as computer supplier and troubleshooter, cheerleader, photographer, proofreader, and so many other roles. I love you.

As always, I am deeply grateful to my parents Fathi Osman (RIP) and Aida Osman, my first introducers to aspects of the *yamas* and *niyamas*, albeit within a different framework. I would not be where I am now without them. Finally, this book would not have been possible without the clients from whom I learned invaluable experiences, and who have allowed me the honor of being with them on their journeys. Thank you for guiding me throughout the years.

Introduction

My psychotherapy client John (not his real name) was telling me about the anxiety that he had been experiencing lately.

"Where do you feel that anxiety?" I asked.

John was perplexed. "What do you mean?"

"What sensations in your body tell you that you're anxious?"

"Oh," John replied. "I don't feel it in my body. I feel it in my mind. I have all these racing thoughts."

I invited John to close his eyes and scan his body. How did his legs feel? His belly? His chest?

"Wow," John responded, surprised. "Now I get what you're asking. My legs feel kinda heavy. I have butterflies in my stomach. My chest feels tight, like it's hard to breathe."

I explained to John that emotions are not only related to thoughts, but also to physical sensations. At some level, we are aware of that. We talk about "butterflies" in our stomachs at times of nervousness or excitement, tightness in our chests at times of sadness, and tension in our shoulders at times of stress. We talk about "holding our breath" during moments of suspense.

But like John, most of us have not been trained to notice our physical sensations until they become overwhelming. Instead, we pay attention to the thought and the story. If we notice anger, we replay in our minds the argument that we had. As a result, we get ourselves more worked up as we focus on that moment in the past when the argument occurred, instead of noticing the signs of anger in the body that we have in the present. Even when we try to shift how we're feeling, we do that by attempting to change the thought – by endeavoring to replace it with a more uplifting one or repeating a positive affirmation – rather than by being with and ultimately moving through the physical sensation.

As far back as the 1880s, William James, dubbed the "Father of American Psychology," argued that emotion is the mind's conceptualization of physical sensation. In other words, we feel something physically, and our mind assigns it an emotion. We sense an elevated heartbeat, and our mind calls that fear. "What kind of an emotion of fear would be left," James argued,

> if the feeling neither of quickened heart-beats nor of shallow breathing, neither of trembling lips nor of weakened limbs, neither of goose-flesh nor of visceral stirrings, were present ... Can one fancy the state of rage[,] and picture no ebullition in the chest, no flushing of the face, no dilation of the nostrils, no clenching of the teeth, no impulse to vigorous action, but in their stead limp muscles, calm breathing, and a placid face?

Therefore, James elaborated,

> *If we fancy some strong emotion and then try to abstract from our consciousness of it all the feelings of its bodily symptoms, we find we have nothing behind,* no "mind-stuff" out of which the emotion can be constituted, and that a cold and neutral state of intellectual perception is all that remains.
>
> (James, 1961, p. 246; italics are James's)

Since James, there have been debates within the field of psychology that place different emphases on the cognitive and physical aspects of emotion. But physiological changes are clearly at least a major aspect of emotion. As neuroscientist Antonio Damasio (2005) points out, "Many of the changes in body state – those in skin color, body posture, and facial expression, for instance – are actually perceptible to an external observer." In fact, Damasio highlights, the very etymology of the word *emotion*, which literally means "movement out," implies an external direction from the body.

As far back as the 1940s, psychologist Nina Bull noted that "any behavior ... requires some postural preparation" (Lewis, 2012, p. 46). For instance, if I ask you to demonstrate depression, you might slump your shoulders and hollow out your chest. For anger, you might tense your body, ball your fists, and scrunch up your face. Now, in one of these positions, think of something that typically makes you happy, and notice how easy it is to feel that. Not so easy, right? We can see that our body language reflects our sense of self, and a connection between open body posture and mood has been supported by several psychological studies (Duclos et al., 1989; Riskind, 1984). As Liebler and Moss (2009) note in their book *Healing Depression the Mind-Body Way*, "What a story a slumping body tells about its overburdened mind!" (p. 163).

A few years ago, in a set of five experiments, 701 participants were presented with a series of stimuli that elicited different emotions. After each stimulus, they were asked to color on a silhouette the regions where they felt sensations. Participants consistently associated different emotions with distinct locations of sensation in the body. And significantly, across different cultural contexts, people colored the same regions when they felt the same sensations (Nummenmaa et al., 2014).

Yet despite all this, the rest of the body continues to be overlooked in the treatment of mental and emotional health. Even our more recent talk of "the mind–body connection" implies that we are linking two separate things, as if the mind were distinct from, rather than a part of, the body. Even though we can acknowledge that illness in much of the body tends to be accompanied by low spirits and cognitive dullness, and that physical activity is key in supporting emotional health, for some reason we still evaluate emotional health separately from other realms of physical health.

In working with their clients, therapists typically pave the path to mental well-being through talk therapy, accessing emotions via thoughts instead of – rather than in addition to – physical sensations. Focusing on thoughts can certainly help us gain insight into a suitable course of action. But insight doesn't necessarily bring about change. How many times have you or someone you have known been aware that you needed to make a change of some sort, but been unable to find the motivation to do it?

Along similar lines, has someone ever told you to calm down when you've been anxious or angry? And did you calm down when they said that? Usually, the answer is no. That thought to "calm down" doesn't end up changing the physical sensation of anxiety or anger, and can in fact lead to more frustration and irritation. Deeper involvement directly with the body is often necessary. For example, if you extend your exhale, that stimulates your parasympathetic nervous system, which is associated with "resting and digesting," and therefore you may feel a little calmer in the moment.

This is especially the case if you have experienced trauma, which is often an underlying trigger for emotional health imbalance. In trauma, the frontal lobe, associated with reasoning, shuts down, and the limbic system, linked with emotions, takes over. As a result, trying to truly deal with trauma through reason is basically impossible, and the fact that many trauma survivors have physical symptoms indicates that trauma is "remembered" in the body (West et al., 2017). As well-known psychologist and yoga teacher Bo Forbes (2011) explains, *"Conceptual insight is not required for change; in some cases it actually interferes with it.* By working in a body-based realm, we can bypass this mental interference. We can *feel* rather than *think* the emotional experiences that heal us" (p. xiii).

The rise of yoga, somatic psychology, and body psychotherapy is indicative of our society's deep need to stretch beyond the cognitive for psychological healing. Over the past two decades, millions in the West have been turning to yoga as a healing modality. As argued by renowned psychiatrist Bessel van der Kolk (2015), "yoga [is] ... a terrific way to [re] gain a relationship with the interior world, and with it a caring, loving ... relationship to the self" (p. 273). Father of American psychology William

James noted over a century ago that those practicing yoga showed "strength of character, personal power, unshakability of soul." In the 1930s, one of the earliest researchers into yoga in the United States, Kovoor Behanan (1938) of Yale University, described yogis as "a group which, through continuous psychological and physiological practices, achieves and maintains a state of emotional stability" (p. 240).

So, what is yoga? If you are someone who is new to it, you might think of yoga as a physical activity that emphasizes flexibility. You may have images of "bendy" people contorting themselves into some pretzel-like shape. While postures like that can be part of a yoga practice, this book is not about fancy poses. There are no inversions, arm balances, or poses that require unusual flexibility.

More importantly, physical poses are not the essence of yoga. Yoga is not about outward form at all; rather, it's about what is going on inside a person. Derived from the Sanskrit word *yuj*, which means "to unite or integrate," the word "yoga" refers to the harmonizing of the body with the mind and breath, and essentially means "that which brings you to reality."

One succinct yet enlightening description is that of researchers Butzer, LoRusso, Shin, and Khalsa (2017), who described yoga as "a comprehensive system of practices for physical and psychological health and well-being." They outline four key components of a yoga practice:

- Physical postures/exercises to promote strength and flexibility.
- Breathing exercises to enhance respiratory functioning.
- Relaxation strategies that focus on reducing tension and stress.
- Meditation/mindfulness practices to enhance mind–body awareness and improve attention and emotion regulation skills (p. 605).

Yoga helps to build physical strength, flexibility, and balance. But it also helps to build *psychological* and *emotional* strength, flexibility, and balance. According to the central classical texts of yoga, the *Yoga Sutras*, yoga is "the stilling of the fluctuations of the mind" (*Sutra* 1:2). One way that the non-stop fluctuations and chatter of the mind – including negative self-talk and self-doubt, which are key aspects of emotional distress – can be calmed is through a focus that is outside that mind chatter, such as via the physical movement or breath of yoga.

Another thought that comes to mind about yoga is that it is a religion. While yoga in its original formulation is certainly spiritual, as practiced in the West it takes many forms, ranging from the fully secular to the deeply spiritual. Often in the West the emphasis is on its "many benefits to the physical and emotional health of practitioners" (Brisbon & Lowery, 2011, p. 934). As Pilkington and her colleagues succinctly summarize, "It can be practised [*sic*] secularly and has been used clinically as a therapeutic intervention" (Pilkington, Kirkwood, Rampes, & Richardson, 2005, p. 15).

The following is an experiment that would help most of us to be able to feel some of the physical and mental/emotional shifts that can happen with less than one minute of yoga. However, just because I mentioned that it helps most of us feel some effects, this does not mean that you have to feel anything, or that you are doing it wrong if you do not feel something. One of the most important things that make a yoga practice a *practice* and not a series of exercises is how you meet yourself. We'll talk about this more in Chapter 1, under the title "witness consciousness."

Come to a standing position, with your feet hip-width apart, arms by your sides. If standing is difficult for you, you can do this sitting in a chair, also with your feet hip-width apart. Close your eyes. What would be the first word that comes to mind that describes how you feel? Do not think about it too hard or doubt your instinct – just go with the first word.

Now we will do a movement called the breath of joy. It has four steps. The first three all involve taking a quick breath in through the nose, and then the fourth step involves exhaling forcefully, so that your breath makes a "ha" sound, through the mouth. If you have unmedicated high or low blood pressure or you are pregnant, you don't want your breaths to be as forceful. Just make them 50% of your maximum forcefulness.

Step 1: Swing your arms up so they're at shoulder level, directly in front of you, while inhaling quickly through the nose.

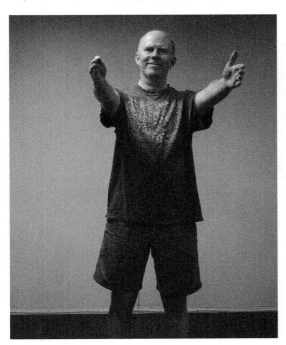

Figure 0.1

Step 2: Swing your arms out so they're at shoulder level, in a T-position, while inhaling a second time quickly through the nose.

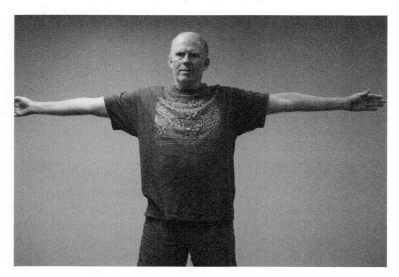

Figure 0.2

Step 3: Swing your arms overhead, while inhaling a third time quickly through the nose.

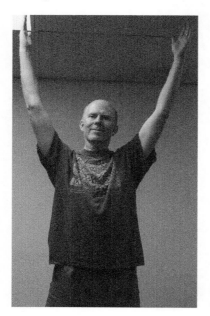

Figure 0.3

Step 4: Exhale forcefully through the mouth with a "ha" and bend all the way forward, so that the crown of your head is reaching down towards the floor. If you are sitting in a chair, bend your torso forward so that it hangs between your knees. If you have unmedicated high or low blood pressure or you are pregnant, make sure that your breaths aren't as forceful, and also only bend forward till your torso is parallel to the floor (i.e., at no more than 90 degrees from your legs if you're standing).

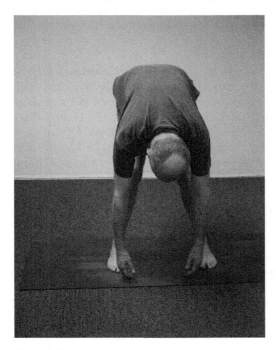

Figure 0.4

Come back up, and repeat this breath three more times. As you become more familiar with it, allow yourself to move through it faster if that is comfortable for your body. It's not a big deal if you do not get the order of the arm movements quite right. After the fourth round, close your eyes and notice what is going on. What would be the first word that comes to mind that describes how your body feels? Again, don't think about it too hard or doubt your instinct – just go with the first word. Just make sure that it describes how your *body* specifically feels.

Did the breath shift anything in you? If it did, notice what that was. If it did not, notice that too. It is not better or worse to feel a shift – you are simply running an experiment to see the effect of different yoga practices on your body. If there has been a shift, it can show up in a variety of ways. You may feel happy, excited, balanced, grounded, angry, agitated, or sad. Now and throughout all the practices in this book, any shift or non-shift that you notice is fine. Your yoga practice (including your response to it) is your own, not a one-size-fits-all experience.

In 2012, the U.S. National Health Interview Survey revealed that 9.5% of U.S. adults (21 million) turned to yoga to address health issues (Clarke et al., 2015), making it the top mind/body practice used for that purpose. This was a significant increase from 6.1% in 2007 and 5.1% in 2002. In 2016, a comprehensive study (Yoga Alliance, *Yoga Journal*, & the Ipsos Public Affairs, 2016) revealed that of the 36.7 million Americans practicing yoga that year, 37% reported starting yoga and 35% continuing it specifically for mental health benefits. In addition, 56% reported starting yoga and 53% continuing it for stress relief.

If Americans are coming to yoga for mental health benefits, then the person guiding their practice needs to be comfortable working with these concerns. While there is now more overlap between the worlds of psychotherapy and yoga than there has ever been before (cf. Forbes et al., 2011; Weintraub, 2015), the gap is still wide. Whenever I train yoga teachers and yoga therapists on emotional health concerns, I ask at the start how many feel trepidation about the subject matter of the course. Without fail, at least half raise their hands.

This response is reflective of the views of society at large, often due to the stigma surrounding mental health as well as the myth that people with mental health diagnoses are violent and unpredictable. In fact, the vast majority are no more likely to be violent than anyone else – only 3%–5% of violent acts can be attributed to individuals living with a serious mental illness (Stuart, 2003). And in reality, since we all are human beings with emotions, that means that there is a mental health component to every client story – we just often choose not to see it or address it directly.

As opposed to yoga therapists who are unfamiliar with mental health, psychotherapists may be unfamiliar with the role of yoga within it. They may recommend "stress relieving activities" such as yoga without a solid idea of how they function, what to expect, and how to work with them. Sometimes they are yoga practitioners themselves, and assume that general population yoga classes will provide their clients with the same relief that they themselves have experienced, or that even another client with similar symptoms has experienced. Yet, just as talk therapy differs from a casual chat, and instead involves specific goals, interventions, and contraindications, so a therapeutic yoga session is distinct from a general population yoga class in the same manner. While researchers on the effects of yoga on emotional health warn that "there may be risks to engaging in yoga" and advise that "healthcare providers can help patients evaluate whether a particular community-based yoga class is helpful and safe for them" (Uebelacker & Broughton, 2016), in fact, most mental health practitioners are unprepared to do so and often unaware that such a step may be necessary.

While a few titles exist on limited aspects of yoga and mental health, there is no overarching work — as yet — that provides an overview of yoga, mental health, research on the intersection of the two, and a step-by-step formulation on how to work with yoga for mental health purposes. This book meets that need. The objective of the volume is to provide a client-centered, step-by-step approach to healing for those experiencing anxiety, depression, bipolar, trauma-related, obsessive-compulsive disorder (OCD)-related, psychotic, and personality disorders, as well as addictions, eating disorders, and attention deficit hyperactivity disorder (ADHD). The book focuses on the experiential as well as the scholarly, since it is impossible for us to truly internalize a method unless we ourselves have experienced it.

The primary audience for the book is psychotherapists and yoga therapists, who are directly addressed throughout. However, an important secondary audience is individuals struggling with mental health diagnoses, and their families, who can benefit from the practices provided here. If you are a psychotherapist, you will encounter some information about mental health conditions with which you are deeply familiar. I would suggest that you still read through it, as it is presented in a way that will then be related to the central framework of the book. Also, reading through those sections can serve as what in yoga we call "beginner's mind" (approaching an experience as if it were brand new and noticing its details with a fresh eye). Similarly, as this book is intended for the seasoned practitioner of yoga as well as the beginner, if you are in the former category, there will be information about yoga with which you are familiar. I would suggest that you nonetheless read through that section, for the same reasons.

This book is made up of eight chapters and a conclusion. The information given about yoga, mental health, and the research on the intersection of the two is — while hardly comprehensive — still relatively thorough, which means that you might find yourself reading parts of it in stages. Just like when eating a sandwich (an analogy that we will encounter again later), feel free to take bite-sized portions, chewing each well to digest it before moving to the next.

Chapter 1, titled "Understanding Yoga," sets the foundation for the book. It outlines some basic elements of yoga: relevant aspects from the eight limbs of yoga (e.g., ethics, postures, breathwork, and meditation) and related themes of yogic philosophy (states of mind, mental afflictions, levels of consciousness, and non-attachment). From this foundation, the chapter moves on to introduce the centerpiece of this book: the Three-Pronged Model that I have developed for working with mental and emotional health. This model presents both the professional and the lay practitioner with an easy and safe step-by-step individualized framework. Based on my experience of hundreds of client case studies, the model begins with a focus on grounding practices, and then — if, and only if, appropriate — moves either to practices that increase vitality and build energy (Sanskrit *brahmana*) or practices that are soothing and calming (Sanskrit *langhana*).

Chapter 2, "Understanding Mental/Emotional Health," provides an overview that is both an informative introduction for the newcomer to this field (e.g., the yoga instructor and the client) and a helpful review of core relevant information for the seasoned mental health professional. It includes an overview of anxiety, mood, trauma-related, obsessive-compulsive-related, psychotic, and personality disorders. The chapter begins to tie the central Three-Pronged Model to some of these diagnoses, thus starting to train the reader in how to apply the model and discern the potential direction of care within it.

Chapter 3, "How Yoga Affects Mental/Emotional Health," provides an accessible overview of some of the research that has been carried out on the effect of yoga on mental health. Just in the last few years, dozens of articles have been published on the subject. The chapter distills key findings from that growing body of research and uses these to further contextualize the Three-Pronged Model.

Building on the relevant background information on yoga, mental health, and research findings, Chapter 4, "Beginning the Practice," is the first chapter in the application portion of the book. It guides the professional through the main points to consider before, at the start of, and throughout working with a client on emotional health.

Chapters 5, 6, and 7 explore the Three-Pronged Model in depth. Chapter 5, "Grounding and Creating Presence," discusses the starting point for any client with a mental/emotional health concern: grounding, stabilizing poses. The chapter also describes other instances in which such a practice continues to be appropriate. Chapter 6, "Building Energy and Vitality," focuses on the next category of poses that may be adopted after grounding has been established – ones designed to build energy and vitality (*brahmana* practices) – outlining the contexts in which these would be used. Chapter 7, "Calming and Soothing," focuses on the other category of poses that may be adopted after grounding has been ascertained – ones designed to calm and soothe (*langhana* practices) – providing the contexts in which these would be appropriate. It also discusses calming practices that specifically build focus – for ADHD, for example.

Each of Chapters 5, 6, and 7 provides an easy-to-follow system of practices that are appropriate for its respective category, including thoughtfully selected physical poses, breath practices, visualizations, and meditations. The chapters guide the professional to begin slowly in order to meet the client where she is, and then gradually transition to practices that help the client build at her own pace and according to her own physical and emotional comfort and needs. Variations are given for postures so that the professional can work to the client's physical ability. If you are reading this book for your own self-help, this can be a guide for which practices may be helpful for you. Each of the chapters ends with a vignette about a challenging situation that arose for me at some point when working within that category, and how I chose to approach it.

Chapter 8, "Working with Addictions and Eating Disorders," expands the use of the Three-Pronged Model to provide a strategy via which to assess how to use the model in these contexts, intake specific to addiction work, and a plan on how to progress in the practice. Again, variations are given for each posture so that the practitioner can work to the client's physical ability.

The conclusion sums up the main points of the Three-Pronged Model and its application, and points to avenues for further exploration.

There a few additional points that I would like to highlight about working with this book. First, I have attempted to combine a degree of readability with a certain level of comprehensiveness. This means that at times it may seem that the information included is too dense to read through in one sitting, and at others it will strike you that the material is not thorough enough for your purposes. Certainly feel free to focus on the material that you need, and supplement the information provided with additional resources as appropriate.

Second, this book is not meant for treatment of children. Treatment of children requires a different approach due to variations in brain chemistry and plasticity, as well as the challenges of self-report as the main source of data for progress.

Third, you should consult with a physician before starting any program.

Finally, I must emphasize that this book should serve as a complement to whatever treatments you are already receiving. If you are a yoga teacher or yoga therapist, under no circumstance should you suggest to your client to take a break from his medication or psychotherapy, or imply to him that yoga will be the miracle cure. That would be irresponsible and unethical, and outside your scope of practice and competence. If you are the person on medication, never stop taking it or shift treatment without consulting a medical professional. Rather, the aim is to provide yoga as an *additional* tool that can help you in your journey towards mental and emotional health.

Mental health and wellness are the key to living a satisfying, meaningful life, and I am grateful that you have chosen to pursue them with the help of this book. I do hope that this book serves you on your journey, whether it is your own or someone else's that you are guiding and witnessing.

References

Behanan, K. (1938). *Yoga: A scientific evaluation.* New York, NY: The Macmillan Company.

Brisbon, N. M., & Lowery, G. A. (2011). Mindfulness and levels of stress: A comparison of beginner and advanced hatha yoga practitioners. *Journal of Religion and Health, 50*(4), 931–941. doi: 10.1007/s10943-009-9305-3

Butzer, B., LoRusso, A., Shin, S. H., & Khalsa, S. B. (2017). Evaluation of yoga for preventing adolescent substance use risk factors in a middle school setting: A preliminary group-randomized controlled trial. *Journal of Youth and Adolescence, 46*(3), 603–632. doi: 10.1007/s10964-016-0513-3

Clarke, T. C., Black, L. I., Stussman, B. J., Barnes, P. M., & Nahin, R.L. (2015). *Trends in the use of complementary health approaches among adults: United States, 2002–2012. National Health Statistics Reports, 10*(79), 1–16. www.cdc.gov/nchs/data/nhsr/nhsr079.pdf

Damasio, A. (2005). *Descartes' error: Emotion, reason, and the human brain.* London, UK: Penguin Books.

Duclos, S. E., Laird, J. D., Schneider, E., Sexter, M., Stern, L., & Van Lighten, O. (1989). Emotion-specific effects of facial expressions and postures on emotional experience. *Journal of Personality and Social Psychology, 57*(1), 100–108. doi: 10.1037/0022-3514.57.1.100

Forbes, B., Akhtar, F., & Douglass, L. (2011). Training issues in yoga therapy and mental health treatment. *International Journal of Yoga Therapy, 21,* 7–11. http://boforbes.com/wp-content/uploads/2013/07/BoForbes-Training-Issues-in-Yoga.pdf?9e2dc7. Accessed April 6, 2018.

James, W. (1961). *Psychotherapy: The briefer course.* G. Allport (Ed.). New York, NY: Harper Torchbooks.

Lewis, D. J. (2012). Nina Bull: The work, life and legacy of a somatic pioneer. *International Body Psychotherapy Journal, 11*(2), 45–58. www.ibpj.org/issues/articles/Daniel%20J%20Lewis%20Pages%2045-58%20IBPJ%20Vol.11,No2_v1c.pdf. Accessed April 14, 2018.

Liebler, N., & Moss, S. (2009). *Healing depression the mind-body way.* Hoboken, NJ: Wiley Publishing.

Nummenmaa, L., Glerean, E., Hari, R., & Hietane, J. K. (2014). Bodily maps of emotions. *Proceedings of the National Academy of Sciences of the United States of America, 111*(2), 646–651. doi:10.1073/pnas.1321664111

Pilkington, K., Kirkwood, G., Rampes, H., & Richardson, J. (2005). Yoga for depression: The research evidence. *Journal of Affective Disorders, 89,* 13–24. doi: 10.1016/j.jad.2005.08.013

Riskind, J. H. (1984). They stoop to conquer: Guiding and self-regulatory functions of physical posture after success and failure. *Journal of Personality and Social Psychology, 47*(3), 479–493. doi: 10.1037/0022-3514.47.3.479

Stuart, H. (2003). Violence and mental illness: An overview. *World Psychiatry, 2*(2), 121–124. www.ncbi.nlm.nih.gov/pmc/articles/PMC1525086/. Accessed April 14, 2018.

Uebelacker, L. A., & Broughton, M. K. (2016). Yoga for depression and anxiety: A review of published research and implications for healthcare providers. *Rhode Island Medical Journal, 99*(3), 20–22. doi: 10.1176/appi.focus.16104

van der Kolk, B. A. (2015). *The body keeps the score: Brain, mind, and body in the healing of trauma.* New York, NY: Penguin Books.

Weintraub, A. (2015). Yoga and mental health: The crumbling wall. In E. G. Horovitz & S. Elgelid (Eds.), *Yoga and mental health: Theory and practice* (pp. 161–171). New York & London: Routledge.

West, J., Liang, B., & Spinazzola, J. (2017). Trauma sensitive yoga as a complementary treatment for posttraumatic stress disorder: A qualitative descriptive analysis. *International Journal of Stress Management, 24*(2), 173–195. doi:10.1037/str0000040

Yoga Alliance, *Yoga Journal*, and the Ipsos Public Affairs. (2016). *2016 yoga in America study.* www.yogaalliance.org/Portals/0/2016%20Yoga%20in%20America%20Study%20RESULTS.pdf. Accessed April 14, 2018.

Part I
Background

1   Understanding Yoga

Relieving suffering is the focus of the practice of yoga, making its lens an invaluable one via which to view emotional health. To better appreciate that perspective, we will survey the origins, development, and central philosophy of yoga. This will give us a context in which to understand the Three-Pronged Model I have developed to work with emotional health, which I will be introducing at the end of the chapter. If yoga and its philosophy are unfamiliar to you, do not be daunted: you can begin to work with the Three-Pronged Model while you are in the process of familiarizing yourself with some of this information. The yoga practices in this book are rooted in movement and breathwork; the rest of the information presented enriches the practice at many levels, but can be explored gradually.

The Origins and Development of Yoga

The Origins of Yoga

While the earliest existing documentation of yoga is in the Rig Veda, an Indian text believed to have been written between 1700 and 1100 BCE, in general, today's yoga is based on the *Yoga Sutras* of Patanjali, a work dating from 200 to 300 CE that is believed to be a collection of earlier materials (Brisbon & Lowery, 2011; Coward, 2002). Based on the Sanskrit word *sutra*, meaning "thread" (from which is derived English "suture") and referring to "threads of wisdom," the *Yoga Sutras* offer guidelines for living a meaningful and purposeful life. The *Yoga Sutras* fell into obscurity until the late 19th century, when they gained popularity thanks to the efforts of Indian teacher Swami Vivekananda (1863–1902), to whom we will return shortly.

The classical texts describe yoga as a form of mental rather than physical discipline, with four paths: *jnana yoga* (the path of wisdom or intellect), *bhakti yoga* (the path of devotion, and love of God and others), *karma yoga* (the path of mindful action and service to others), and *raja yoga* (the path of encountering and transcending the thoughts of the mind via meditation).

Hatha yoga – the physical yoga to which we are accustomed in the West – has traditionally been considered preparation for *raja yoga* (Bahadur, 1977; Connolly, 2007).

The emphasis on *hatha yoga* in India began in earnest in 1933, when the palace in the state of Mysore hired Tirumalai Krishnamacharya (1888–1989) to run its yoga hall. A scholar of Sanskrit, Ayurveda medicine, and other classical disciplines, Krishnamacharya is hailed as the "Father of Modern Yoga," as he sequenced yoga postures, combined them with deep breathing, and generally led the way for both becoming an integral part of yoga, instead of a step towards meditation. Furthermore, Krishnamacharya produced a number of gifted students, including B.K.S. Iyengar, K. Patabhi Jois, and T.K.V. Desikachar, respectively the developers of the styles of Iyengar, Ashtanga, and Viniyoga, which have become so popular in the West (Broad, 2012; Mohan & Mohan, 2011).

History of Yoga in the West

While raja yoga had gained significance in the West from the 1880s among groups such as the Theosophical Society (Ervast, 1921), more general Western awareness of yoga and meditation came with the World Parliament of Religions, held in Chicago in 1893. The Parliament marked the first time that Western audiences on American soil received spiritual teachings from South and East Asian teachers. Swami Vivekenanda – the Indian teacher who had popularized the *Yoga Sutras* – came to the United States to present at the Parliament, and then went on to teach meditation practitioners in New Hampshire and established ashrams (places of spiritual retreat) around the country (Taylor, 1999). Just over two decades later in 1920, Paramahansa Yogananda arrived in the United States as India's delegate to an International Congress of Religious Liberals, founded the Self-Realization Fellowship (SRF) to disseminate his teachings on yoga and its tradition of meditation, and also began lecturing around the country.

The Immigration Act of 1924 limited the number of immigrants allowed entry into the United States, leading Westerners to travel East to seek teachings. In 1947, Indra Devi, the first Westerner to study with Krishnamacharya and the first to bring his lineage to the West, opened a yoga studio in Hollywood. Her three popular books brought *hatha yoga* to the demographic with which it now tends to be associated in the West: women. In 1950, Richard Hittleman returned from studies in India to teach yoga in New York, presenting a nonreligious physically oriented yoga for the American mainstream that even came to be featured on television (De Michelis, 2005).

A confluence of major events half a century later led to an even broader awareness by many Americans of at least the existence of yoga. The 1960s, with their counter-culture movements and exploration of alternate world views, alongside circumstances leading to an influx of Asian spiritual teachers to the West (Taylor, 1999), served as a catalyst for the spread of yoga-related teachings. Outside of the political realm, a central factor leading to yoga gaining a boost in the United States was the recognition of its benefits, first for fitness and second for countering stress. From this grew yoga's association with emerging forms of complementary and alternative medicine (De Michelis, 2005).

Yoga in the West Today

Now, in the United States, there are dozens of types of yoga, often named after a key teacher or concept. Different styles of yoga are characterized by variations in posture and breathwork practice. As Richard Rosen (2015) highlights, it's more appropriate to think of the term "hatha yoga as an umbrella term than as a monolithic praxis" (p. 25). For instance, the three styles of yoga originated by Krishnamacharya's three students, B.K.S. Iyengar, K. Patabhi Jois, and T.K.V. Desikachar, differ dramatically in terms of emphasis and pacing, highlighting the creativity within the yoga tradition.

But despite the variation in the particulars of the practice, from the second half of the 20th century on, yoga classes in the West – whether at a gym, a community center, or a studio, or prerecorded – came to be relatively standardized into an overall structure. That structure can be divided into three parts: introductory quietening time, practice proper, and final relaxation (De Michelis, 2005, p. 251):

(i) "introductory quietening time: arrival and settling in"

For a few minutes at the start of the class, practitioners are typically invited to begin focusing inwards, and to notice their body, breath, and/ or thoughts. They are encouraged to put aside the obligations and roles of their day-to-day lives, and be with their experiences in the immediate moment.

(ii) "practice proper: instruction in postural and breathing practice given by the instructor through example, correction, and explanation"

Depending on the style and the teacher, this segment of the class may involve flowing from one posture to the next or holding poses; the incorporation of a good deal of breathing practice, or not very much; and a focus on a physical theme (e.g., the back), a psychosocial theme (e.g. gratitude), or no particular focus. This section takes up most of the time of the class, typically around an hour.

(iii) "final relaxation: pupils lie down in *savasana* ('corpse pose') ... possibly with elements of visualization or meditation"

Savasana, or corpse pose, is so named because it is a pose of complete stillness that serves as an opportunity to integrate all that preceded it. Practitioners typically lie on their backs in *savasana* for two to ten minutes. They are then slowly guided out, and usually invited to observe any state changes. They may notice a decrease in the fluctuations of the mind, the natural turbulence of their thoughts, and/or the restlessness of the body compared with at the start of their practice.

Basic Tenets of Yoga

Now that we know a little about the development of yoga, we will turn to some of its basic tenets. These give us a template via which to understand mental and emotional health, and will both contextualize and directly inform the model that is at the center of this book. First, we will discuss some practices that are typically explicitly mentioned in a yoga class, and then we will move on to a few other aspects of philosophy.

The Eight Limbs of Yoga

I was first introduced to yoga at my gym in 1997. After class, I got in my car and, as I always did, automatically turned on the radio. But immediately, I found myself turning it off. The radio was interrupting an unusual sense of calm and peace that I was experiencing. As I kept practicing yoga, I continued to be pulled in to that stillness each time I finished a class. But my practice involved only the physical form of *asana* for years, before I came to understand yoga on a deeper level. And honestly, if the physical had not been my path in, I probably never would have come to yoga – it would have felt too alien to me, especially at a time when it had not mainstreamed in the same way that it has in the last couple of decades.

A physical practice was of great benefit to me at the beginning. But physical postures practiced without an eye to the other aspects of yoga can lead to a practice that is superficial, harsh, and ego-based. While I felt a sense of calm after yoga, I would often try to push through poses. At times I was carried away by how a pose looked on the outside, rather than the effect that it had on the inside. But ultimately, yoga is about the inner journey. If I raise my level of anxiety by thinking I need to force myself into a particularly challenging physical form, that does not help my emotional health, however impressive it may be to my ego.

The eight limbs (*ashtanga*) of yoga contribute to that inner journey, and each can be seen as a branch to mental and emotional healing. As we discuss them, some might feel too foreign to you, and that is completely understandable. I am mentioning them now so that if you are unfamiliar with them, you have a chance to know that there are many ways in which you can work with yoga to reach more emotional balance, and that the majority of them do not involve binding yourself into a pretzel. In fact, "by definition, yoga is seen as the control of the five senses and a reduction of mental activity" (Mehta, 2010, p. 157); the physical is simply one way to get there. In this book, we will be learning ways to use two of those limbs in particular – postures and breath – to calm the turmoil that tends to dwell in the mind.

What do we mean by control of the five senses? Most of us tend to look outside of ourselves for fulfillment. Our awareness and energies are directed outward, leading us to believe that we will be happy if we have the right job, relationship, or figure. Yet even when we get the job, the relationship, or the figure that we thought held the key to our happiness, we discover that we are not fulfilled. Our minds continue to chatter with frustration and self-doubt, and our bodies remain restless.

When we experience turbulence of thoughts and restlessness of body, we often look outside of ourselves for a "fix." We may eat, drink, spend hours online, play videogames, or shop. But all these are quick "fixes" that don't fix anything at all. They are distractions. Once they are over, we are back to where we were, and in need of more distraction. Again and again, our experiences show us that nothing external can really shift the internal, yet most of us continue to grasp at the external.

Yamas *and* Niyamas *(Ethics)*

The first two limbs, the *yamas* and the *niyamas*, are the ethics of yoga. *Yama* refers to ethics regarding the outside world, while *niyama* refers to those of the inner world. The *yamas* and *niyamas* are central to a genuine, present-focused, and therefore emotionally healthy practice.

The five *yamas* – nonviolence (*ahimsa*), truthfulness (*satya*), nonstealing (*asteya*), right use of energy (*brahmacharya*), and non-greed (*aparigraha*) – allow us create a yoga practice that helps us develop an inner sense of calm. For example, violence and nonviolence are not just about hurting someone physically, but also emotionally. And if I do not want to hurt someone else emotionally, why would I want to hurt myself? Why would I, for example, want to force myself into a movement that does not work for my body, or berate myself for how I am not able to do a pose "right"? Those are both actions that raise anxiety. The same applies to being true to myself by practicing what works for me (*satya*), not competing with anyone else to produce a pose that brings attention away from them and to myself (*asteya* and *aparigraha*), and using my energy in the wisest way (*brahmacharya*). When I follow these principles, my physical practice will feel smoother.

The same goes for the *niyamas*: cleanliness (*saucha*), contentment (*santosa*), focused energy (*tapas*), study of the sacred scriptures and of one's self (*svadhyaya*), and surrender to God (*Isvara pranidhana*). *Saucha* can be viewed as removing impurities in general. That refers literally to coming to practice with a clean body (who wants to practice next to someone who has not showered?), as well as with a pure mind that does not easily resort to judging others practicing around us or criticizing ourselves harshly. We can also see how approaching our practice with contentment (*santosha*) and focused energy (*tapas*) is helpful, and that being well-informed via study of texts and of one's self (*svadhyaya*) is very useful.

Isvara pranidhara (surrender to God) will sit differently with each of us. For some of us, surrender to God is very natural, and it might be a surprise to know that it is part of the yoga tradition. For others, the concept might feel unfamiliar and even unpleasant. Regardless of where you fall in the spectrum of belief in a "higher power" (to borrow 12-step program language), one of the things that most of us are comfortable with is "being in the zone." "Being in the zone" means that as you practice something, rather than forcing it, it just flows. A cyclist might start a ride pedaling furiously, but at some point he does not have to try so hard; the pedaling comes naturally. A writer may start by plotting out a story, but then at some point her story "writes itself."

Remembering all the pieces of the *yamas* and *niyamas* is in itself a formidable task that can feel overwhelming. For our purposes here, the most important thing to consider is that you are the best judge of where your body needs to be at any given moment, and that taking the time to notice this is the foundation of an authentic practice. If you are leading a practice, check in with your client and yourself. We are all human, and sometimes it can be tempting to push your agenda rather than focus on the needs of the client. If you are leading and your client is not following, whether literally or energetically (e.g., they are doing the poses, but they're not really "into it"), really take the time to listen to them, whether they are sharing something with you verbally or non-verbally. Practice *ahimsa* by not pushing them, *satya* by being true to what they need, and *brahmacharya* by using their energy and yours appropriately. And practice *Isvara pranidhara* by letting go of your ego as a teacher.

If you are the student, really notice how you're feeling in the moment, and be clear with your teacher if you're not ready to go where he is leading you. Resist putting him on a pedestal. He may be knowledgeable, but he will never know your inner experience as you do.

Asana *(Postures)*

The third limb, *asana*, refers to the physical postures that we in the West think of when we hear the word "yoga." But while flexible bodies are usually the first image we have of yoga, traditionally the word "*asana*" refers to a "seat," as the purpose is to prepare the body for meditation (Dalal, 1991). More recently, *asana* has developed to encompass the held poses and fluid movements popular in contemporary yoga classes.

Patanjali defined *asana* only in outline, as it was learned from a *guru* and not from description. That highlights how *asana* is a practice, not a destination. One of the most important things to remember about *asana* is that how a pose appears on the outside is not any indication of whether a person is practicing yoga effectively. I can place my foot behind my head and lead observers to think that I am a great yogi. But if my mind is focused on how impressive I look, I am not really practicing yoga, as I am caught up in how I will be perceived by others and not my inner experience. On the other hand, I can be in a simple seated position and be completely present. Then I am practicing yoga.

When I started practicing yoga, I knew nothing about the *yamas* and *niyamas*, and as a result, my yoga practice was like a building without foundation: it might have looked appropriate on the outside, but it was in danger of cracking internally. I was pushing myself into movements, rather than allowing myself to arrive there. Allowing rather than pushing gives us a practice that is kinder and gentler, more emotionally balanced, and more connected with our true selves. As we read in the *Yoga Sutras* (2:47), "It is through *relaxation* of effort and meditation upon the infinite that asana is perfected" (emphasis mine).

People often think they need flexibility to practice yoga. In fact, if a beginner's body is too flexible, the strength required for certain poses may be a challenge, and that person needs to develop more stability around the joint areas. In this book, we are working with poses that are accessible to the average person. We do not need complicated practices in order to steady, invigorate, or calm the body and mind.

Pranayama (*Breathwork*)

Human beings are the only creatures who have some control over their breath, and we see the connection between breath and mood in day-to-day life. Scholar of religion Marcel Eliade pointed out: "the respiration of the ordinary man is generally arrhythmic; it varies in accordance with external circumstances or with mental tension." For example, "the respiration of a man in anger is agitated, while that of one who is concentrating (even if only provisionally and without any yogic purpose) becomes rhythmical and automatically slows down" (1954, pp. 56, 57).

That control of the breath is the fourth limb of yoga, referred to as *pranayama*. "*Prana*" is "life force," as exemplified in the breath, and "*ayama*" refers to expansion. As we might know from taking deep breaths at times of stress, expansion of the breath can clear physical and emotional obstacles in our body. As noted in the 15th-century *Hatha Yoga Pradipika*, "When Prana moves, the mind also moves" (Bernard, 1968, p. 47).

When we are comfortable and breathe more smoothly, we shift away from the sympathetic to the parasympathetic nervous system, focusing on "rest and digest" rather than "fight or flight." Psychiatrist Bessel van der Kolk (2015) relates the story of a client with high levels of anxiety due to sexual trauma. When he encouraged her to try yoga, what made an immediate impact on her was *pranayama*. She shared with him:

> The teacher ... said that if we notice our breath we are in the present because we can't breathe in the future or the past. It felt so amazing to me to be practicing breathing in that way ... like I had been given a gift.
>
> (p. 278)

Along similar lines, founder of LifeForce Yoga Amy Weintraub (2012) presents the case study of a psychologist's introduction of a yoga breathing practice during her first session with a highly anxious client, in order to provide the client with a felt sense of how she actually had more control than she believed.

Not only does noticing breath keep us in the present and highlight our communication with our bodies, but different methods of using the breath lead to emotional shifts. Just as we will work with *asana* in a variety of ways in this book, we will do the same with *pranayama*.

Pratyahara (*Withdrawal of the Senses*)

The 10th-century philosopher Vachaspati emphasized, "Pranayama renders the mind fit for concentration, by making it steady" (Bernard, 1968, p. 47). Making breathing rhythmical and intentional shifts attention away from outside stimuli to internal experience. This takes us to the fifth limb of yoga, *pratyahara*, the withdrawal of the senses (i.e., sight, hearing, and touch) from the distraction of the outside world, or as Eliade prefers to translate the term, the "ability to free sense activity from the domination of external objects" (1954, p. 68). A teacher in a yoga class might encourage students to practice *pratyahara* by noticing sounds outside the yoga room and then releasing them from focus, thereby creating space for inner experience.

The yogi who finds that his mind is able to "detach" itself from external stimuli in this manner is now ready for the final three limbs, collectively known as *samyama* (integration): *dharana* (concentration), *dhyana* (meditation), and *samadhi* (enlightenment). If, as you are reading this, you are thinking that these last three limbs sound too esoteric for you, know that focus on the first five limbs can bring about remarkable shifts, and that they are the emphasis of the practices in this book.

Dharana (*Concentration*)

Remember the last time you were totally focused and immersed in an activity? Whether it was something creative like painting or writing, or something physical like dancing or running, your mind was still except for attention to that one thing. This state of focus is *dharana*, total concentration on a single point.

The word *dharana* comes from the root *dhr*, meaning "to hold." Swami Vivekananda called the mind "a drunken monkey" (Behanan, 1938, p. 217). *Dharana* holds that drunken monkey to a fixed point that may be internal, like a part of the body or the breath, or external such as a picture, candle flame, or sound. The nature of the object of focus is not so important; the purpose is to quiet the mind with this total concentration, so that there is less room for the turmoil with which the mind tends to occupy itself. As we concentrate our minds, any time other thoughts come up (and they will, very frequently), we simply return our focus to that original point.

Dhyana (Meditation)

Once we are able to concentrate on an object, we can hold that concentration for longer and turn inward. This is *dhyana*, the Sanskrit term for meditation, which literally means "moving through the mind." This is the essence of yoga: the stilling of the fluctuations of the mind (*Yoga Sutra* 1:2 *Yogas chitta vritti nirodha*).

In the West, we tend to think of meditation as an outward form, often a cross-legged position. In fact, meditation is an inner journey. And because we are a "quick fix" culture, when we notice the challenge of calming our minds we tend to dismiss ourselves as candidates for meditation, not realizing that the path to stillness is long for all meditators. As Jon Kabat-Zinn (2003) observes, like any sort of practice, this is an art form that one develops over time, and it is greatly enhanced through regular, daily, disciplined practice.

Samadhi (Enlightenment)

Samadhi occurs when a practitioner, in continuous meditation upon an object, loses all sense of separation between it and himself, and becomes one with it (Coward, 2002). In its transient form, this can be what we think of as a "trance" state, and as we practice more, it may generalize and permeate our lives. We no longer find ourselves caught up in the trappings of like, dislike, judgment, worry, and fear. As we go through our daily tasks, we are no longer prisoners of the melodramatic cycle of mind chatter, replaying the past or agonizing about the future. Rather, we are immersed in the enjoyment of each moment. We still have desires, such as hugging our loved ones or enjoying food, but we are no longer controlled or driven by them.

While this is a highly appealing state, my aim with this book is more humble. I am hoping that by tasting some of the shifts that come with the first four limbs of yoga, you will experience – at least for an instant – a mode of being in the present that takes you out of the typical mind chatter. As psychiatrist Elizabeth Visceglia (2015) notes,

> Educating clients about Yogic concepts such as nondualism, equanimity, nonharming, attention to the present moment, and restraint from judgment can contextualize and deepen important psychotherapeutic insights. These philosophical concepts can be reinforced by the wisdom that emerges from ongoing attention to the breath, the body, and the mind, just as they were by Yogis thousands of years ago.
>
> (p. 153)

The benefit of that for emotional health is invaluable.

Other Aspects of Practice

Supporting the limbs of yoga are other practices that you might encounter in a yoga class, and that we will be referring to at times in this book.

Mudra *(Seal/Gesture)*

A *mudra* is a symbolic gesture often performed with the hands and fingers, although occasionally involving the entire body. Using *mudra*s helps calm and focus the mind, two essential components in working with yoga for emotional health. Many of us are familiar with the gesture where a person brings his palms together in front of his chest (sometimes referred to in the West as "prayer position," since it is the same hand gesture used in Christian prayer). This is referred to as *anjali mudra* (*anjali* is a Sanskrit word meaning "to offer" or "to salute").

Mantra *(Utterance)*

Traditionally in Sanskrit, but sometimes in English, a *mantra* is an utterance (sound, syllable, word, or group of words) that is often used as a concentration point. In a yoga class, a teacher may ask students to focus on the Sanskrit phrase *"Soham"* or its English translation "I am That," perhaps thinking "so" on the inhale and "ham" on the exhale. This may help them regulate their breaths, and have a point on which they can concentrate and therefore calm their minds.

Bhavana *(Imagery)*

Imagery can be used in a variety of ways in a yoga practice. Like *mantra*, it is often used to help the mind focus. For example, if I were guiding you through Mountain pose (described in Chapter 4), I might say, "Imagine yourself as a solid mountain," which may help you access more stability in the pose. After practicing your pose "on the mat," that visualization of the mountain may be one that you bring up at other moments "off the mat," that is, any time throughout your day when you wish to access solidity and stability.

Sankalpa *(Affirmation/Intention)*

In a yoga class, *sankalpa* is often used in the context of setting an intention for that day's practice. The teacher may either suggest the intention or invite students to come up with their own. It may be physical (build more flexibility) or psychosocial (give and receive love). Notice that even the physical is not only physical: if I need flexibility, my mind may also crave it, not just the rest of my body.

Chakras *(Energy Centers)*

In yogic philosophy, there are seven main energy centers throughout the body, generally corresponding to nerve centers. A nerve center is a group of closely connected nerve cells that act together in the performance of some function in the body. Each of these energy centers, or *chakras*, is associated with a location, color, and other characteristics that affect psychological and emotional well-being. The seven principal chakras are:

First/Root *Chakra*, located in the base of the spine in the tailbone area, and related to survival issues such as financial independence, money, and food. It is associated with the color red.

Second/Sacral *Chakra*, located in the lower abdomen, about two inches below the navel and two inches in, and related to creativity, well-being, pleasure, and sexuality. It is associated with the color orange.

Third/Solar Plexus *Chakra*, located in the upper abdomen in the stomach area, and related to self-worth, self-confidence, and self-esteem. It is associated with the color yellow.

Fourth/Heart *Chakra*, located in the center of the chest just above the heart, and related to love, joy, and inner peace. It is associated with the color green.

Fifth/Throat *Chakra*, located in the throat, and related to communication and self-expression of feelings and truth. It is associated with the color blue.

Sixth/Third Eye or Brow *Chakra*, located in the forehead between the eyes, and related to intuition, imagination, wisdom, and the ability to think and make decisions. It is associated with the color indigo.

Seventh/Crown *Chakra*, located at the top of the head, and related to connection to spirituality. It is associated with the color violet, or sometimes with the color white, as it combines all the other colors.

In yoga classes, connections are often made between *asanas* and *chakras* (e.g., emphasizing the first *chakra* while holding Mountain pose). Sometimes, a teacher may use a *chakra* as the theme of a class. For instance, she may focus a class on building love, and lead students through a series of practices related to the fourth/heart *chakra*. In this, she may incorporate *asanas* that move the chest, such as backbends, *mudra*s where the student is touching the heart, such as *anjali mudra* ("prayer position"), and *bhavana/* imagery related to giving and receiving love.

Witness Consciousness

Probably the most valuable long-term learning that comes from a typical yoga class is that of witness consciousness, a concept I briefly mentioned in the Introduction. Witness consciousness basically entails becoming a neutral observer of your own life. In my yoga classes, I often ask students to notice how a pose has affected their bodies. How does the right side of the body feel after the pose? How about the left side? The upper body? The lower body? The front of the body? The back of the body? They may feel differences in some of these areas, and they may not.

It is easy to arrive at a judgment based on what we notice, thinking perhaps if we do not discern any difference that the posture failed. Witness consciousness, however, is by its definition a *neutral* observation of the body. I invited you to practice it in the Introduction to this book, after practicing the breath of joy. I mentioned that you may have noticed a difference after doing the breath, or you may not have. Both those options are fine. It does not mean that the pose failed if we do not perceive a difference. Rather, we simply notice that, and move to the next practice, without judgment or attachment to outcome.

One of the most significant gifts of yoga is a development of witness consciousness in our day-to-day lives. If I as a therapist am working with a client, and I ask that person how she felt after last week's session, my ego leads me to prefer a positive answer over a negative one. I would rather hear "I felt great" than "I felt worse than before." If I am approaching the situation with the eye of witness consciousness, however, my client's answer would lead me to pay closer attention to how I am designing the session and guiding my client, rather than take me down the path of rebuking my client or myself for what I then decide to call a "failed" session. A scolding of my client might include the thought or even spoken words, "Well, perhaps you didn't try hard enough," while a berating of myself might include the thought, "You screwed up." Neither of these is even an accurate assessment; each is simply a guess generated as a response to a situation with which my ego was uncomfortable. Practicing witness consciousness is invaluable both to the student and to the teacher.

Earlier, we mentioned *Sutra* 1:2 – Yoga is the stilling of the fluctuations of the mind. Expanding on that is *Sutra* 1:12: "The fluctuations are stilled by dedicated practice and nonattachment" (*abhyasa vairagyabhyam tan nirodha*). Witness consciousness is a crucial entryway to non-attachment. We practice, and we let go of outcome.

Yoga Philosophy

In addition to the tangible elements that may be part of a yoga practice, we will discuss five other aspects of yoga philosophy that provide a helpful lens through which to view mental and emotional health. These are: *samskaras*, *koshas*, *kleshas*, *gunas*, and states of mind.

Samskara *(Impression)*

In yogic philosophy, every action or intent by an individual leaves a *samskara* (impression, impact, imprint, or groove) in the person's deeper structure. Therefore, thoughts and actions directly relate to a person's sense of suffering, happiness, and contentment.

Koshas *(Sheaths)*

Koshas are sheaths around the body, starting from the periphery and moving towards the core of the self. Each relates to a different aspect of ourselves.

Annamaya Kosha *(the Physical Body)*

This is the outside layer of the body, and refers to the physical body – our muscles, bones, ligaments, and tendons. This *kosha* is most people's motivation to begin a yoga practice, as they wish to increase physical flexibility, strength, and/or balance.

Pranamaya Kosha *(the Energy Body)*

One of the major benefits of yoga is that we become conscious of our breathing, and – sometimes for the first time as adults – we learn to take deep breaths. That generally affects our energy and helps us feel more present.

Manomaya Kosha *(the Mental Body)*

We use the body and the breath to shift the activity of the mind. For example, if you are experiencing chronic anxiety, a calming yoga practice can help shift related feelings and thoughts, thus possibly alleviating some of the anxiety.

Vijnanamaya Kosha *(the Wisdom Body)*

Grounding in the wisdom body gives us a broader perspective on our life experience. For instance, we might come to see that what is causing our anxiety is not actually related to the present moment. With awareness, the anxiety fades. Over time, as we practice yoga, we find ourselves connecting to a deeper level of intuition and greater internal wisdom.

Anandamaya Kosha *(the Bliss Body)*

As we continue to practice, we move beyond distress derived from difficult moments in the past and fears about the future, and into feelings that encompass and include all, such as compassion, love, and joy. Over time, rather than occasionally feeling bliss, we *become* the bliss. That is *Anandamaya kosha*, which may be thought of not as an ecstatic happiness or even joy, but as a steady state of being, no matter what circumstance arises.

Most of us have a tendency to "live" in one kosha over the others. Most Westerners tend to be mind-oriented (in *Manomaya kosha*), but some are body-oriented (in *Annamaya kosha*). However, as Amy Weintraub points out, restriction in one *kosha* tends to lead to restriction in others. "If there is tightness in the chest, for example (anamaya kosha)," Weintraub explains, "the breath may be affected (pranamaya kosha) and there may be a corresponding emotion or mood state (manomaya kosha), and perhaps a belief about the self or the world (vijnanamaya kosha)" (2015, p. 169). Practicing *pranayama* may loosen sensation in the chest, which then affects the other *kosha*s as well. In this way, yoga helps us to balance our awareness of all layers of the Self.

Kleshas *(Obstacles)*

Another of the important elements in yoga philosophy is the concept of *kleshas*: obstacles, afflictions, or "veils" that obscure the truth from us and are the cause of our suffering.

Avidya *(Ignorance)*

The first of the *kleshas*, *avidya* (ignorance), is the root of all the others. It refers to our lack of awareness and disconnection from what is true. For example, when something difficult happens, we may create a story about how things like that always happen, and how they will never change. We begin to speak in absolutes (using "always" or "never," for instance) that are not true. In other words, we're mistaking the impermanent for the permanent. Or we can get caught up in aspects of our identity, thinking that they are our core self. For instance, we may get too caught up in what our job says about who we are, or are deeply crushed when we lose our job because we feel like we are nothing. Instead of seeing the job as something we do and from which we derive meaning, we actually see it as our self. In other words, we mistake the non-self for the Self.

Asmita *(Ego)*

Related to that is the second affliction, *asmita* or the Ego. This is what makes us forget the true limitations and scope of our identities. It can hurt us and others by labeling ourselves as grand and them as substandard in some way. Or we can think we are the ones who are inferior, and they are the superior ones. We may look around and see ourselves as smarter, more accomplished, or more beautiful than those around us, or as stupid, incapable, or ugly compared with someone else. Either way, thoughts like that bring (and mask) intense pain and disconnect us from others.

Ego can also hurt us in more subtle ways. It can make us think that we have more control than we do, and that we need to step in at times that are beyond human capability. For instance, sometimes mental and emotional imbalances develop because we think we should have been able to control a situation that we could not possibly have controlled. Survivors in families where there was abuse can develop anxiety and/or depression due to guilt that they were unable to stop abuse that happened to a younger sibling, even though there was no way as a child that they could have done anything to stop it.

If you were to complete the sentence "I am _____," what would you insert there? Whatever goes in the blank is a label of some sort, and a label is a judgment. For example, a couple of decades ago, probably the first word I would have put in there would have been "smart." But then I went from an educational experience where I was a big fish in a small pond to one where I was a little fish in a big pond, and I did not feel so smart. My egoism and ignorance (mistaking the non-self for the Self) landed me in a depression, and that was actually what started me on my yoga path. Every time since then when I have experienced emotional imbalance, I have noticed that it is because I have made a label an identity and mistaken it for the Self.

Raga *(Attachment)*

The third *klesha*, *raga*, is about attachment, which we mentioned briefly earlier when talking about *Sutra* 1:12: "The fluctuations are stilled by dedicated practice and nonattachment." We are all attached to something. Most of us in this day and age are attached to a cell phone. How disturbed do you feel when you discover that you forgot your cell phone at home? Does it throw off your day, or are you able to take a step back and notice what it's like to create some space between you and that phone? If you are, then you are able to lift the veil of *raga* (attachment) a little through the experience of witness consciousness.

We are not only attached to things – we also become attached to outcomes. We can have expectations about how things in our lives will turn out, and when they do not go that way, we can experience intense emotional imbalance. When health circumstances led me to make an unforeseen professional shift, I was seriously rattled. My identity had been wrapped up in my profession, I had mistaken the non-self for the Self, and I had been deeply attached to a life story in which I remained in that professional context for the rest of my career. "We feel that we have something to gain or lose if a certain situation develops one way or another," yoga scientist Kovoor T. Behanan (1938) explained, and so "we become identified with the emotion" (p. 116). We can see *avidya*, *asmita*, and *raga* all at work here.

Some days, our bodies move smoothly. We flow from one pose to the next effortlessly. The following day, we return to the same sequence, and it seems more challenging. We can become frustrated, but if we are not attached to the outcome, we can meet ourselves where we are in the moment. This is sometimes referred to as "beginner's mind," which means that we are doing everything as if it were the first time we were doing it. Think of a baby playing with her feet and laughing joyfully as she curiously explores. This is now our exploration as adults.

Many people, when they hear that attachment is an obstacle to liberation and that we are working towards non-attachment, worry that their life will become joyless. Does non-attachment also mean that we will not be attached to those whom we love? But non-attachment in relationships is not indifference or apathy to another person. It is an absence of fear and clinginess, so that we can focus on the actual person, not the dread of losing them and the ensuing limitations that creates.

Dvesha *(Aversion)*

Just as we can become attached to things and stories, we can also have inflexible narratives about what we do not want. We reject certain people, habits, and options without giving them a chance. I did this about meditation when I was in my early twenties. A friend asked me if I meditated, and I right away responded, "That's not my thing." And now look what happened! If I had clung to that particular aspect of my veil of *dvesha*, or aversion, my life would have turned out very differently.

"We perceive as good that which brings pleasure … we perceive as bad that which brings pain," explains Jaganath Carrera in *Inside the Yoga Sutras* (2006, p. 105). On the mat in a physical yoga practice, this can translate into dislike of a certain pose. We may say, "I hate backbends," because they are uncomfortable for us. But if we really sit with why we do not like them, we might find out that they are uncomfortable psychologically, not physically. Perhaps doing one will be a lesson in stepping outside our comfort zone, to new ground.

You may feel that you do not tend to do that, and that instead you jump into everything eagerly, enthusiastic to meet new adventures. In that case, ask yourself what it would be like to challenge yourself and hold back a little. Do you feel an aversion to that?

Abhinivesha *(Clinging to Life)*

The fifth klesha is *abhinivesha*, or clinging to life. It is a rare person who lives life with an openness towards death: most of us are afraid. We become "mesmerized by the distractions and attractions of the world," describes Carrera, "and become reluctant to vacate the premises" (2006, p. 113).

I used to do psychotherapy work with hospice clients. They would be given a terminal diagnosis and be terrified of death. Then, as time went on, sooner or later, they would accept it, and a shift would happen. Suddenly, there would be what felt like a decrease of turbulence, and at times even what looked like an increase of energy, to the extent that those close to them would think that their loved one was getting better. But the energy comes from releasing that clinging to life. It would also make me think: if we released our clinging to life earlier in our life span, would we be able to tap into that energy earlier?

As we shed the *kleshas*, we move towards *viveka*, which can be translated as "right understanding" or "discernment." It is the ability to differentiate between some of the concepts described: the real and unreal, eternal and temporary, Self and non-Self, pleasure and bliss. At times in this book, I will urge us to notice when we are becoming pulled into "the story" (of mistaking the unreal for the real), and urge us towards that discernment.

Gunas *(Qualities)*

The concept of *gunas* directly informs the model that is the core of this book. *Gunas* are qualities that form the essential aspects of all nature. The three *gunas* are:

Sattva: illumination through comprehension, radiance, and luminosity. When *sattva* predominates, consciousness is calm, clear, comprehensible, and virtuous.
Rajas: motor energy, mental activity, and passion. If the mind is in *rajas* it is agitated, uncertain, and unstable, experiencing the world as chaotic, confusing, and demanding.
Tamas: obscurity, lethargy, static inertia, and heaviness. If the mind is in *tamas*, it will be lazy, depressed, and demotivated, experiencing the world as dark and confusing (Eliade, 1954).

We each have a predominant *guna*, which acts as a lens that affects our perceptions of and perspective on the world around us. At the same time, the mind's psychological qualities are unstable and can quickly fluctuate between different *gunas*. It is tempting to want to be in *sattva* frequently, as it forms the base for many positive attributes, but attachment to that outcome is still an attachment, and it can lead to its own maladaptive states (Sullivan et al., 2018).

States of Mind

The *guna*s contribute to the states of mind, of which there are five:

Ksipta *(Restless)*

Have you ever found yourself unable to focus? I would be surprised if you said "no," as most of us experience a version of this at some time or other. This is what we refer to in yoga as "monkey mind" – remember Swami Vivekananda's analogy of the mind as a "drunken monkey?" – where a person is highly agitated and unable to think, listen, or keep quiet.

The *ksipta* mind is overcome by the *rajas guna*. You can imagine that if you felt like this more often than not, it would get in the way of day-to-day functioning.

Mudha *(Torpid)*

Sometimes, the opposite is the case. We feel sluggish and slow moving. Just today, a friend said she was looking for her keys. I could see them on the counter, but my mind did not make the connection between her words and what I was seeing. The mind in *mudha* is dull and listless, and no information seems to reach it.

The *mudha* mind is overcome by the *tamas guna*. You have probably felt this way sometimes too. And again, while some of us occasionally feel it, others do so frequently that it starts getting in the way of living a smooth life.

Viksipta *(Distracted)*

Viksipta describes a state of distraction that may be caused by several factors, including sickness, doubt, carelessness, lethargy, or worldliness. These distractions may cause pain, dejection, restlessness of the body, and unsteadiness of the breath (*Yoga Sutras* 1:31). Again, we are all distracted at times, but some of us are consistently so, especially in cases when we have experienced trauma. Distraction is not only about being "scattered;" it can also show up as dissociation or numbness.

Ekagra *(One-pointed)*

This is the first of the two states of mind towards which we are working in yoga. In *ekagra*, the mind is in a state of relaxed attention. *Ekagra* can be achieved via *asana*, where the body is concentrated in a single position (Eliade, 1954), or *pranayama*, where it is focused on a breath. This is why yoga classes will sometimes incorporate a meditation at the end, after *asana* or *pranayama* have led practitioners to this state.

Nirodha *(Mastered)*

Once the mind is in a state of relaxed attention, it is not distracted by random thoughts, and can be fully absorbed in the object of focus. Yogic practices transform our mental agitation (*vritti*), emotional wounds (*samskara*), and false identifications (*gunas*) towards a state of acceptance (Kreher, 2015).

Bringing It Together: The Three-Pronged Model

Now that we have a basic understanding of some aspects of yogic philosophy, we can move on to a discussion of the Three-Pronged Model, which may be applied in working with any mental health condition. The man hailed as the "Father of Modern Yoga," Tirumalai Krishnamacharya, was known for his statement, "Teach what is appropriate for an individual" (Mohan & Mohan, 2011, p. 38). That is the aim of this model, which presents the therapist and the client with an easy and safe step-by-step case conceptualization.

In a recent issue of *Yoga Journal* (November 2017), senior yoga teacher Natasha Rizopoulos explains:

> Many of us have a tendency toward one end of the energetic spectrum. Those who are industrious and inclined toward action are sometimes too goal oriented and attached to results, while those who are more relaxed and easy going can fall prey to lassitude and lack persistence in their efforts. Each of these extremes can lead to an agitated mind: Chasing after specific ends can produce a disturbed or restless psyche, while the inability to commit to a course of action can make for a scattered and distracted mind.
>
> (p. 52)

We can recognize here the states of *ksipta* and *viksipta*, as well as the potential for *mudha*. Rizopoulos expands: "Like so many things in yoga, the solution is to find a path that is less binary, where opposites can coexist and balance each other" (p. 52).

This is where the core of the Three-Pronged Model comes in. Within the Ayurveda tradition (yoga's sister science of health, which literally means "knowledge of living"), there exist two energetic principles: *brahmana* and *langhana*. *Brahmana* is "that which builds/expands," and *langhana* is "that which lightens/reduces." These two energetic principles can be thought of as similar to the yin and yang energies of Chinese medicine, with one being invigorating and the other calming. The idea is that we can lean on these two principles and tailor our practice to the energy shift we need. But before exploring *brahmana* and *langhana*, it is imperative to work with grounding.

Grounding

Grounding is the first and most essential prong of the Three-Pronged Model. If we are not centered and grounded, and are instead in the distraction of *viksipta*, an emotional shift may be too much for us in that moment. In some cases, grounding may be all we use, as it might be unsafe to do anything else. In Chapters 2 and 5, I will explain when and why that might be. One can be eager to jump into deeper practices that are touted to create more rapid shifts, but that can be harmful. Every client needs first to start with grounding work, and only transition from there once grounding has been clearly established.

Grounding emphasizes balance and evenness. In *asana*, this means maintaining straight lines, symmetry, and contact with the floor on both sides of the body, if this is available physically. In *pranayama*, it means maintaining the same breath count on the inhale and exhale, and breathing in and out through the nose. We will talk more about this in Chapter 5.

Brahmana

Brahmana refers to practices that increase vitality, and energize the body and mind. *Asanas* that encourage *brahmana* energy may include back movement in the spine, movement in the hips, and invigorating flow between movements. *Pranayama* breathing that increases *brahmana* includes breaths with a long inhale and a rapid, more forceful exhale, such as what we encounter in pulling *prana* (see Chapter 6), or even just a longer inhale and shorter exhale (please do not try this yet, as it can lead to hyperventilation if not done correctly). Only when a client presenting in a *mudha* state is appropriately grounded do we incorporate *brahmana* practices. We will talk more about this in Chapter 6.

Langhana

Langhana refers to soothing practices. Yoga *asanas* and breathing that promote *langhana* relax the body, reduce the heart rate, stimulate the parasympathetic nervous system, and calm the mind. *Asanas* that encourage *langhana* include forward bends and restorative styles, while *pranayama* breathing includes breaths with a longer exhale than inhale. And similarly, only when a client presenting in a *ksipta* state is appropriately grounded do we incorporate *langhana* practices. We will talk more about this in Chapter 7.

A general population class may combine elements of *brahmana* and *langhana* practices, or focus on one over the other. However, when we experience imbalance, we can have so much *rajas* or *tamas* that a general practice may perpetuate our lack of equilibrium. We may need more *langhana*, but if we go to a class that includes *brahmana* and *langhana* equally, it is as if we have one pile with five jellybeans and another with three, and keep adding an equal number of jellybeans to each one. The pile with five will always have more, as it started out with more. We have to add more to the pile with three in order for them to equalize.

Or, some of us may lean into our imbalance, and practice in a way that further exacerbates it. For example, if we are experiencing *rajas* we may favor a *brahmana* practice, as slowing down is too emotionally challenging for us. As we keep turning to this active practice, sooner or later, we burn out and are out of balance even more. That is another reason why we need a customized practice that meets us where we are, and gradually builds from there towards the shift we need.

The Three-Pronged Model is an efficient, easy-to-use template for working with others or yourself. However, it is not a magic prescription. It took time for any of us to arrive where we are emotionally, and it will take time to shift. You may quickly experience a state change (a shift during the moment you are practicing), but it may take a while to notice a trait change (a shift that you perceive at other times throughout your day). But regardless of when your conscious mind starts becoming aware of them, the changes are happening as you embark on your therapeutic yoga journey.

I look forward to being with you on that journey.

References

Bahadur, K. P. (1977). *The wisdom of yoga: A study of Patanjali's Yoga Sutra*. New Delhi, India: Sterling Publishers Private Limited.

Behanan, K. (1938). *Yoga: A scientific evaluation*. New York, NY: The Macmillan Company.

Bernard, T. (1968). *Hatha yoga: The report of a personal experience*. New York, NY: Samuel Weiser.

Brisbon, N. M., & Lowery, G. A. (2011). Mindfulness and levels of stress: A comparison of beginner and advanced hatha yoga practitioners. *Journal of Religion and Health, 50*(4), 931–941. doi: 10.1007/s10943-009-9305-3

Broad, W. J. (2012). *The science of yoga: The risks and the rewards*. New York, NY: Simon & Schuster.

Carrera, J. (2005). *Inside the Yoga Sutras: A comprehensive sourcebook for the study & practice of Patanjali's Yoga Sutras*. Buckingham, VA: Integral Yoga Publications.

Connolly, P. (2007). *A student's guide to the history and philosophy of yoga*. Sheffield, UK: Equinox Publishing.

Coward, H. (2002). *Yoga and psychology: Language, memory, and mysticism*. Albany, NY: SUNY Press.

Dalal, A. S. (1991). *Psychology, mental health & yoga*. Twin Lakes, WI: Lotus Press.

De Michelis, E. (2005). *A history of modern yoga: Patanjali and Western esotericism*. New York, NY: Bloomsbury Academic.

Eliade, M. (1954). *Yoga: Immortality and freedom*. (W. Trask, Trans.). Kingsport, TN: Kingsport Press.

Ervast, P. (1921). *The mission of the theosophical society: An open letter to theosophists the world over*. Helsinki, Finland. http://media.pekkaervast.net/penet/books_files/ The_Mission_of_the_Tehosophical_Society.pdf. Accessed April 5, 2018.

Kabat-Zinn, J. (2003). Mindfulness-based interventions in context: Past, present, and future. *Clinical Psychology: Science and Practice, 10*(2), 144–156. doi: 10.1093/ clipsy.bpg016

Kreher, S. (2015). Yoga for anger management. In E. G. Horovitz & S. Elgelid (Eds.), *Yoga therapy: Theory and practice* (pp. 172–184). New York & London: Routledge.

Mehta, P., & Sharma, M. (2010). Yoga as a complementary therapy for clinical depression. *Complementary Health Practice Review, 15*(3), 156–170. doi: 10.1177/ 1533210110387405

Mohan, A. G. & Mohan, G. (2011). *Krishnamacharya: His life and teachings*. Boulder, CO: Shambhala Publications.

Rizopoulos, N. (2017, November). Practice well: Embodying the Sutra. *Yoga Journal*, p. 52.

Rosen, R. (2015). Yoga history and philosophy in the West. In E. G. Horovitz & S. Elgelid (Eds.), *Yoga therapy: Theory & practice* (pp. 22–31). New York & London: Routledge.

Sullivan, M. B., Erb, M., Schmalzl, L., Moonaz, S., Taylor, J. N., & Porges, S. W. (2018). Yoga therapy and polyvagal theory: The convergence of traditional wisdom and contemporary neuroscience for self-regulation and resilience. *Frontiers in Human Neuroscience, 12,* 67. doi: 10.3389/fnhum.2018.00067

Taylor, E. (1999). Introduction. In M. Murphy & S. Donovan (Eds.), *The physical and psychological effects of meditation: A review of contemporary research with a comprehensive bibliography 1931–1996*. Petaluma, CA: Institute of Noetic Sciences.

van der Kolk, B. A. (2015). *The body keeps the score: Brain, mind, and body in the healing of trauma*. New York, NY: Penguin Books.

Visceglia, E. (2015). Psychiatry and yoga therapy. In L. Payne, T. Gold, E. Goldman & C. Rosenberg (Eds.), *Yoga therapy & integrative medicine: Where ancient science meets modern medicine* (pp. 143–155). Laguna Beach, CA: Basic Health Publications, Inc.

Weintraub, A. (2012). *Yoga skills for therapists: Effective practices for mood management*. New York, NY: W. W. Norton & Company.

Weintraub, A. (2015). Yoga and mental health: The crumbling wall. In E. G. Horovitz & S. Elgelid (Eds.), *Yoga and mental health: Theory and practice* (pp. 161–171). New York & London: Routledge.

2 Understanding Mental/ Emotional Health

What Is Mental Health?

In the Introduction, we talked about the mind as part of the body. Yet, we are trained to refer to the health of the mind as separate from that of the rest of the body, even though we recognize that mental health affects and is affected by "physical" health. Personally, I prefer to use the term "emotional health" over "mental health," as it describes what we are talking about – the health of the emotions – without trapping us in an artificial mind–body dichotomy. For the next couple of paragraphs you will still see the phrase "mental health," however, as we examine some general understandings of it.

According to the World Health Organization (WHO, 2018a), mental health is

> a state of well-being in which the individual realizes his or her own abilities, can cope with the normal stresses of life, can work productively and fruitfully, and is able to make a contribution to his or her community. Mental health and well-being are fundamental to our collective and individual ability as humans to think, emote, interact with each other, earn a living and enjoy life.

From this we see that mental/emotional health is – as the WHO stresses – "more than just the absence of mental disorders or disabilities." Similarly, in its definition of mental health, Medilexicon's medical dictionary specifies both "the absence of a mental or behavioral disorder" and "a state of psychological well-being in which one has achieved … an appropriate balance of love, work, and leisure pursuits."

When mental/emotional health is out of balance, mood, behavior, and thinking can all be affected. That is when we have what we generally term "mental disorders" or "mental illnesses." The American Psychiatric Association has defined these as health conditions involving changes in thinking, emotion, and/or behavior that are associated with distress and/ or problems with functioning in social, work, or family activities. The changes are not attributable to the physiological effects of a substance or to another medical condition, and symptoms may be continuous or episodic.

Just as I am more partial to the term "emotional health" rather than "mental health," I also prefer to use the word "imbalance" instead of "illness." "Illness" suggests that you are either ill or you are not, whereas "imbalance" implies a range that most of us may feel in some shape or form, at some point in time. My first psychotherapy mentor taught me to view diagnoses on a continuum, which allows us to focus on the humanity of the person, as well as the commonalities we might have with them. I appreciate the literal interpretation of the word "disorder" as "dis-order," highlighting the fact that life is disrupted and out of order, but unfortunately the term "mental disorder" tends to carry a stigma.

Emotional health imbalance is not due to personality weakness or character flaws – people do not "get over it" if they try hard enough. Rather, there are many potential contributing factors, both biological and sociological. The former comprise genetics, brain chemistry, and family history, while the latter may include trauma or abuse, conflict, loss, financial concerns, or medical problems. Even in cases of genetic predisposition, life stress – particularly in the form of adverse experiences in childhood – has been shown to increase an individual's risk. For example, while variations in the serotonin transporter gene have been seen in individuals with depression, those with the vulnerable genotype who are maltreated and raised in an environment without social support tend to have higher rates of depression than those who have adequate social support (Kinser, Bourgignon, Whaley, Hauenstein, & Taylor, 2013). Even positive life events can trigger emotional imbalance, as they may lead to the emergence of new stressors, uncertainty, and questions of identity.

Mental/emotional imbalance is something that affects more people than we think. According to the World Health Organization (2018b), depression is the leading cause of disability in the U.S. for those aged 15–44. According to the American Psychiatric Association, nearly one in five (19%) U.S. adults experience some form of mental illness, one in 24 (4.1%) suffers from a serious mental illness, and one in 12 (8.5%) has a substance use disorder. Nearly half (45%) of those with any mental disorder meet criteria for two or more disorders, and over 8.9 million persons have dual diagnoses – that is, both a mental and a substance use disorder. Mental health and trauma-related disorders are among the top five most costly conditions in the noninstitutionalized population in the United States – alongside heart disease, cancer, and asthma – with expenditures at $57.5 billion and $68 billion a year, respectively (Kinser et al., 2013; Soni, 2009).

Far more significant than the cost in dollars is the cost in lives. In the United States, from 1999 through 2014, the suicide rate increased by 24%, from 10.5 to 13.0/100,000 population. Globally, rates have increased by over 60% in the last 45 years, to 16/100,000. This translates to one person committing suicide every 40 seconds, making the number of people who die by suicide greater than that of people killed annually in crimes or war. The World Health Organization cites suicide as the fourth leading cause of death worldwide, and by 2020 it is expected to be the second. There are indications that for every adult who dies by suicide there may have been more than 20 others attempting it (Tucci & Moukaddam, 2017; World Health Organization, n. d.).

Yet in our society we are not taught how to maintain emotional health. As renowned researcher and yoga teacher Sat Bir Khalsa notes,

> When you went through high school, you were never taught how to deal with stress, how to deal with trauma, how to deal with tension and anxiety – with the whole list of mood impairments. There's no preventive maintenance. We know how to prevent cavities. But we don't teach children how to be resilient, how to cope on a daily basis.
>
> (Broad, 2012, p. 78)

We have not put our collective and individual resources into building an integrated mental health system. Despite defining mental health as more than the absence of illness, our health care resources are nonetheless channeled into treating and caring for mentally ill patients. As a result, by the time clients come to a health provider, they have usually hit a crisis point. It is time for us to focus not on "fixing" emotional imbalance, but on cultivating emotional well-being.

Yoga and Psychology: A Comparison

In Chapter 1, we talked about how yoga, as a holistic system, aims at alleviating suffering. As researcher Victoria Follette notes, yoga and psychotherapy both seek "to foster growth, understanding, and freedom from suffering. Furthermore, both share a fundamental assumption that there is an inherent potential within each person toward continual growth" (Follette, Palm, & Pearson, 2006, p. 48). Marvin Levine (2009) notes several connections between the two areas, including the concern with alleviating inner suffering, the teaching of the appropriateness of compassion, the highlighting of maturing and growth, and the acknowledgment that the mind functions at both a more superficial level and a deeper level that can give rise to a monitoring of thoughts and emotions.

Furthermore, we see additional areas of overlap between yoga and specific therapeutic approaches. Both yoga and psychoanalysis, for example, emphasize the unconscious. While Freudian psychoanalysis focuses on "the darkest, the most perilous, the unhealthiest part of the nature" and in that regard differs significantly from yoga, the work of Jung, who saw yoga as a parallel way of understanding the psyche, is far more similar (Coward, 2002, p. 4; cf. Dalal, 1991). Abraham Maslow's hierarchy of needs also touches on the core of yoga. Beginning with the physiological and culminating originally in self-actualization – described as achieving one's full potential to become the most that one can be – in later years Maslow expanded the hierarchy to include one more level: self-transcendence. "Transcendence," Maslow explained,

> refers to the very highest and most inclusive or holistic levels of human consciousness, behaving and relating, as ends rather than means, to oneself, to significant others, to human beings in general, to other species, to nature, and to the cosmos.
>
> (1971, p. 269)

We can see here the parallels between this view and our discussion about yoga in Chapter 1.

However, there are core differences between psychotherapy and yoga. The most significant is that yoga has a loftier goal than the mental awareness and insight of psychotherapy: to liberate the human being from the shackles of self-doubt and pain. The goal of yoga is not to obtain something that is lacking: it is the realization of an already present reality from which we have become separate (Carrera, 2005). "In Yoga," explains Dalal, "the aim is to attain a progressively more evolved state of being than that of mental consciousness, thereby attaining a progressively greater force of one's being" (Dalal, 1991, p. 56). If we relate this to the *kosha* system, we see that Western psychotherapy tends to focus only on *manomaya kosha* (the mental body), without attention to other *kosha*s.

Within this model, yoga views affliction as an aid to spiritual transformation, and therefore something from which to be learned. In yoga philosophy, "it is the human attempt to 'get rid' of suffering that is false. We cannot toss our suffering aside, we must nourish it ... Yoga, which means 'yoke' or 'unite,' is intended to bring together all aspects of our lives, including our frailty and afflictions" (Douglass, 2011, p. 91). Therefore, "Yogis ... became experts not just at palliation but at pulling up suffering by its roots" (Cope, 2004, p. xii).

As a result of this central divergence between most of Western psychology and yoga, there is a significant difference regarding the view of the interplay between the mind and the emotions. Psychotherapy has traditionally aimed at controlling and overcoming negative emotions; for example, cognitive behavioral therapy emphasizes changing a behavior or thought pattern. Yoga, on the other hand, is not prescriptive in this manner; rather, it is a form of inquiry into how we, as individuals, experience the interplay between our thoughts and our bodies. Yoga researcher and therapist Laura Douglass elaborates on this: "I do not see the yoga classes I teach as 'therapeutic' for my goal is not to provide or assist in a cure" (2011, p. 85).

Some psychotherapeutic models have adopted a "middle way," so to speak, between these two approaches. As recent literature has suggested that the primarily change-based emphasis of cognitive behavioral therapies may be limited (for example, results show that the efficacy of the usual care for depression – pharmaceutical management and cognitive therapy – is poorer than originally thought), mental health practitioners have been advocating for the importance of acceptance and mindfulness in the course of successful psychotherapy (Kinser et al., 2013). For example, dialectical behavioral therapy (DBT), mindfulness-based cognitive therapy (MBCT), and acceptance and commitment therapy (ACT) have been developed to help patients live a more satisfying life while noticing symptoms instead of attempting to control them. These approaches (particularly ACT and DBT) espouse a dialectical world-view in which clients are encouraged to accept where they are in life, while being challenged to act more effectively in the future (Follette et al., 2006).

Even with the development of psychotherapy modalities that highlight noticing rather than "fixing," the body's place continues to be on the fringes of Western psychology. Pioneers in mental health such as Alexander Lowen (d. 2008), who "understood that suppressed emotions, unhappiness, and anger can block energy flow and cause physical distress" (Weintraub, 2015), and that a depressed person was out of touch with his body, have been an anomaly. Even as somatic psychology develops, it is still generally not taught in mainstream psychotherapy graduate programs.

But movement beyond traditional methods is sorely needed, as people turn to complementary and alternative options for symptom relief. As far back as 2001, a total of 56.7% of people experiencing anxiety attacks and 53.6% of those with severe depression reported turning to complementary and alternative therapies. Even among those being treated by a conventional provider, a total of 65.9% of the respondents experiencing anxiety attacks and 66.7% of those with severe depression had resorted to complementary and alternative therapies (Kessler et al., 2001).

My personal experience with clients strongly indicates that yoga is a highly effective adjunct to talk-based therapy. My clients note that their talk therapy was enriched by their yoga practices, which allowed them to be more in the present, make new connections, process body experiences, and sit with emotions more comfortably. They could also utilize yogic postures or breathing techniques from the session at other times throughout their day, to calm themselves during difficult moments and to build a general norm of equanimity.

The Role of Trauma

We mentioned earlier that while there are important biological factors that contribute to emotional imbalance, life stressors are often key. One of the most important things to understand when focusing on emotional health is the role of trauma. Most people with chronic emotional imbalance have experienced some sort of trauma, and practitioners need to understand and be sensitive to this in their work.

An event is traumatic if it is extremely upsetting and at least temporarily overwhelms an individual's inner resources (Telles, Singh, & Balkrishna, 2012). Trauma is generally divided into two categories: single incident and complex. When we think of trauma, what typically come to mind are one-time or single-incident events: natural disasters, mass interpersonal violence, large-scale transportation accidents, house or other domestic fires, motor vehicle accidents, rape and sexual assault, physical assault by a stranger, or victimhood from torture or war.

But based on the preceding definition, anything that overwhelms a person's inner resources is a trauma. Trauma does not need to be large scale, and more often than not, it is not due to one single incident. Listing traumas separately gives the erroneous impression that they exist individually and independently of one another. People may have been exposed to a series of traumas, or they may have been exposed to consistent, long-term trauma. For example, according to research psychiatrist Bessel van der Kolk, for every soldier who is traumatized by war, 30 children are traumatized at home (van der Kolk, 2017).

Which brings us to complex trauma: multiple unresolved traumas with severe, diverse, and persistent impacts. Complex trauma can be caused by circumstances within the family, such as childhood physical/sexual or verbal/emotional abuse, neglect, or family violence or dysfunction; or within the environment, such as structural violence (e.g., attitudes such as racism, sexism, homophobia, or transphobia that are embedded in the general political and economic organization of society and put specific individuals and populations in harm's way), civil unrest, war trauma, genocide, cultural dislocation, or sexual exploitation. An extensive literature review of U.S. Government sources, as well as retrospective and other clinical studies, reports that one out of four girls and one out of six boys is sexually abused before the age of 18. Only 10% of these assaults are committed by strangers; the rest are by parents, siblings, foster caregivers, neighbors, or family acquaintances (Lilly & Hedlund, 2010).

In complex trauma, the stressors typically occur at developmentally vulnerable times in a person's life, and as a result, can lead to serious effects: "changes in the mind, emotions, body, and relationships ... including severe problems with dissociation, emotional dysregulation, somatic distress, or relational or spiritual alienation" (Ford & Courtois, 2009, p. 13). Furthermore, victims of interpersonal trauma tend to be at greater risk of additional interpersonal traumas. For example, those who have experienced abuse as children are more likely to be victimized as adults (Rhodes, 2015; Telles et al., 2012).

It is well recognized that psychological trauma causes impairment of the neuroendocrine systems in the body, with activation in the sympathetic nervous system (associated with fight or flight, as well as freeze) and suppression of the parasympathetic nervous system (associated with rest and digest). There is also an increase in the level of circulating cortisol, which has adverse effects on different body systems. Furthermore, environmental structural trauma such as poverty has been demonstrated to affect the very structure of the brain. In a National Institute of Mental Health longitudinal cohort study of 389 children, reduction in volume of the brain's gray matter, frontal lobe, temporal lobe, and hippocampus were seen (Evans & Kim, 2013; Hair, Hanson, Wolfe, & Pollak, 2015).

When it comes to official diagnoses, people respond to trauma in different ways. Exposed to the same trauma, some may develop posttraumatic stress disorder (PTSD), whereas others may experience symptoms of depression, anxiety, or personality disorders. In some, increased suppression and avoidance may lead to emotional numbing and dissociation, where the person's mind is not fully in the here and now. Some may have physical health problems, such as obesity, heart disease, or chronic pain syndromes. Others may have the milder diagnosis of adjustment disorder or no official diagnosis, but instead extreme self-reliance or chronic feelings of being alone in the world.

Regardless of diagnosis, trauma survivors often live with a chronic stress response of emotional arousal; they are "on high alert" even in the absence of current danger. Their brains are biased towards warning under any circumstances. They may fluctuate between extremes of intrusive reliving of trauma symptoms in their bodies and minds, and conscious or unconscious avoidance of these overwhelming emotions, sensations, and thoughts. Women with complex trauma histories of abuse often feel disconnected from their bodies and struggle to feel secure (Rhodes, 2015). That means that as therapists, we need to hold a safe space and tread lightly. We will talk more about this in Chapter 4.

Some Mental Health Diagnoses

As we just saw, trauma can bring about a variety of imbalances such as PTSD, depression, and anxiety. The rest of this chapter outlines the emotional health imbalances that are most commonly diagnosed in adults, based on descriptors in the Diagnostic and Statistical Manual of Mental Disorders (DSM), the main reference manual used by mental health professionals in the United States. First published in 1952, the most recent edition of this reference text – the fifth edition, and therefore known as the DSM-5 – came out in May 2013.

In presenting some of these diagnoses, I have sacrificed excessive detail for readability, so please remember that I am giving you general information here. If you are a yoga therapist working with a client with a specific diagnosis, I would suggest researching that in greater depth. Also, if you are a yoga therapist, please do not use these descriptors to give a diagnosis to your client, and ensure that a client coming to you with a diagnosis actually received that diagnosis from a mental health professional, rather than solely via their own internet or other research.

Anxiety Disorders

An estimated 40 million U.S. adults suffer from anxiety disorders – roughly 18% of the nation's population. While most of us feel anxiety at some point, what makes it a chronic imbalance is when it gets in the way of a person's day-to-day life. Certainly, most of us experience stress, which may be defined as the pressure that life events – such as work, school, major life changes, or trauma – exert on an individual and the way in which that pressure impacts emotions (Brisbon & Lowery, 2011). But when the immediate stressor is gone yet the emotional arousal remains, this, now, is anxiety. It is important to distinguish between state anxiety, where the feelings of anxiety come and go depending on the circumstances, and trait anxiety, where there is a chronic tendency towards anxiety. While most of us have state anxiety from time to time, "anxiety proneness" is what usually constitutes a diagnosis of an anxiety disorder.

Anxiety disorders share a tendency for the sufferer to have a severe fear that is linked to certain objects or situations, and therefore to avoid exposure to them. The following four disorders are among the most commonly diagnosed:

Generalized Anxiety Disorder (GAD)

When we think of a person as generally anxious, this is the diagnosis for which they might be considered. In GAD, a person has persistent and excessive worry, anticipating disaster about any number of things, including money, health, family, work, or school. Individuals with GAD find it difficult to control their worry, which may seem more than warranted, or they may expect the worst even when there is no apparent reason for concern. Approximately 7 million people a year in the U.S. suffer from GAD.

Panic Disorder

Panic disorder is diagnosed in people who experience panic attacks that occur unexpectedly, and are preoccupied with the fear of a recurring attack. Panic attack symptoms typically include a racing heart; feeling weak, faint, or dizzy; chest pains; breathing difficulties; tingling or numbness in the hands and fingers; and feeling sweaty or having chills. During a panic attack, the person feels a loss of control, and experiences sudden paralyzing terror of imminent disaster. Panic disorder can interfere a great deal with daily life, causing people to avoid situations that they fear might instigate them. The interference is greatest when people also have agoraphobia, an avoidance of places where they feel immediate escape might be difficult. These may be open places (like parking lots) or enclosed places (like theaters). Approximately 3 million people a year in the U.S. suffer from panic disorder.

Social Anxiety Disorder (Social Phobia)

This is the extreme fear of being scrutinized and judged by others in social or performance situations. It is *not* simply shyness. Often people with social anxiety disorder are social and want to connect with people, but cannot. Although they recognize that the fear is excessive and unreasonable, they feel powerless against their anxiety, and are terrified they will humiliate or embarrass themselves. The anxiety can interfere significantly with daily routines, occupational performance, or social life, making it difficult to complete school, interview and get a job, and have friendships and romantic relationships. Approximately 15 million people a year in the U.S. suffer from social anxiety.

Specific Phobias

Phobias are a disproportionate fear of objects (e.g., animals) or situations (e.g., flying, heights, receiving an injection, seeing blood). In the U.S., nearly 8.7% of adults have at least one extreme specific fear, and nearly 25 million Americans report a phobia of flying.

Depressive Disorders

"Depression is the common cold of the deluded human being," yogi and social worker Stephen Cope explains, "[a]nd according to the Buddha, all human beings are quite deluded" (Weintraub, 2004, p. 27). The Centers for Disease Control and Prevention has estimated that depression impacts over 26% of the U.S. adult population, with more than 1 in 20 reporting moderate to severe symptoms (Tucci & Moukaddam, 2017). As we mentioned earlier, it is the leading cause of disability in adults under the age of 45, and the World Health Organization (2012) anticipates that by the year 2030, it will be the biggest health problem on our planet.

In day-to-day speech, we frequently use the word "depressed" when we really mean "sad." We might say, for example, "I was so depressed yesterday morning, but then my friend called and I felt better." Here we are describing a temporary, transient state, a reaction to something sad that we might have experienced. But depression is not transient. It is chronic, and we may continue to feel it even after things around us shift.

There are two main categories of depression — major depressive disorder and persistent depressive disorder — and a few situational types of depression, such as premenstrual dysphoric disorder. Here we'll look at the two more general types of depression.

Major Depressive Disorder (MDD)

In MDD, nearly every day for at least two weeks, a person experiences a minimum of five of the following symptoms: depressed mood or irritability for most of the day; consistent decreased interest or pleasure in most activities; significant weight change (5%) or change in appetite; change in sleep, whether insomnia or hypersomnia; change in activity, whether psychomotor agitation or retardation; fatigue or loss of energy; feelings of worthlessness or excessive or inappropriate guilt; diminished ability to think or concentrate, or more indecisiveness; persistent physical symptoms that do not respond to treatment, such as chronic pain or digestive issues; or thoughts of death or suicide.

MDD can be episodic, although the majority of individuals with MDD experience recurrences, and every recurrent episode increases the probability of another, a phenomenon known as "kindling." MDD has a high rate of comorbidity with other conditions, with anxiety being the most common. MDD significantly affects daily functioning, such that up to 60% of depressed individuals report that the condition has a severe or very severe negative impact on their daily lives (Kinser et al., 2013).

Persistent Depressive Disorder

As opposed to major depressive disorder, where the main feature is the depth of depression, in persistent depressive disorder (previously referred to as "dysthymia") the principal aspect is its chronicity. For the diagnosis, an adult has to have experienced depressed mood for most of the day, for more days than not, for a minimum of two years. At least two of the following are present: poor appetite or overeating; insomnia or hypersomnia; low energy or fatigue; low self-esteem; poor concentration; or feelings of hopelessness. During the two-year period, the symptoms have not been absent for more than two months at a time.

The DSM-5 specifies different manifestations of depression, including with anxious distress (feeling keyed-up or tense, restless, or worried, and fearing that something awful will happen, or that there will be a loss of control) or with melancholic features (loss of pleasure in all or almost all activities, and lack of reactivity to usually pleasurable stimuli). Note the overlap between these manifestations and the *rajasic* (*ksipta*-dominant) or *tamasic* (*mudha*-dominant) modes we discussed in the previous chapter.

Up to half of all women with a diagnosis of depression may experience "anxious depression," typified by repetitive negative thinking about one's depression and life situations (Kinser et al., 2013).

Bipolar Disorders

In a given year, more than 3.3 million American adults (1.7%) suffer from bipolar disorder (Kessler, Petukhova, Sampson, Zaslavsky, & Wittchen, 2012). Bipolar disorder typically begins in adolescence or early adulthood. Contrary to how it is sometimes used in conversation, a diagnosis of bipolar disorder does not mean a person is highly emotional. Rather, it refers to someone who experiences extended periods of mood and energy that are excessively high and or/irritable alongside ones of sadness and hopelessness, sometimes with periods of "normal" mood in between. While everyone experiences ups and downs, the shifts that happen in bipolar disorder are typically severe, are unrelated to the person's day-to-day circumstances, and have a serious impact on a person's life.

There are three main types of bipolar disorder:

Bipolar I Disorder

This is defined by manic episodes that last at least seven days, or by manic symptoms that are so severe that the person needs immediate hospital care. Mania includes excessive energy, activity, restlessness, racing thoughts, and rapid talking (also called "pressured speech"); extreme "high" or euphoric feelings; being easily irritated or distracted; decreased need for sleep; unrealistic beliefs in one's ability and powers, with exaggerated self-confidence or unwarranted optimism; uncharacteristically poor judgment; unusual sex drive or abuse of drugs; provocative, intrusive, or aggressive behavior; and signs of psychosis.

Usually, depressive episodes occur as well, typically lasting at least two weeks. Episodes of depression with mixed features (having depression and mania symptoms at the same time) are also possible.

Bipolar II Disorder

This is defined by a pattern of depressive episodes and hypomanic episodes, rather than the full-blown manic episodes of bipolar I disorder. A hypomanic episode is an emotional state characterized by a distinct period of persistently elevated, expansive, or irritable mood, lasting at least four days. The mood is present for most of the day nearly every day, and it is clearly different from the person's usual mood. Hypomanic episodes have the same symptoms as manic episodes, with two important differences: the mood usually is not severe enough to cause problems in the person's work or socializing with others or to require hospitalization, and there are no psychotic features present during the episode.

Cyclothymic Disorder (Cyclothymia)

In adults, this is defined by numerous periods of hypomanic symptoms as well as numerous periods of depressive symptoms lasting for at least two years. However, the symptoms do not meet the diagnostic requirements for a hypomanic episode and a depressive episode.

Trauma-Related Disorders

As we have discussed, trauma can result in a number of imbalances, including depression and anxiety disorders. However, sometimes it results in psychological injuries that we specifically describe as trauma-related disorders, such as acute and posttraumatic stress disorders.

Acute Stress Disorder

Acute stress disorder refers to a series of symptoms that may have arisen between three days and one month after exposure to actual or threatened death, serious injury, or sexual violation. These symptoms may come from any of the five categories of intrusion, negative mood, dissociation, avoidance, and arousal, which will be explained under PTSD. Acute stress tends to be identified in an average of 20% of cases following traumatic events that do not involve interpersonal assault – ranging from 10% in cases of severe burns to 13–21% in cases of motor vehicle incidents – and in 20–50% of cases of interpersonal traumatic events such as assault, rape, or witnessing a mass shooting (American Psychiatric Association, 2013, p. 284).

Posttraumatic Stress Disorder (PTSD)

Once a person has been experiencing post-trauma symptoms for over a month, they may qualify for a diagnosis of PTSD. While "having PTSD" is yet another term we use relatively indiscriminately, PTSD is a specific psychological injury in which the brain behaves as if the person were still in the trauma-inducing situation. As Shay succinctly summarizes, PTSD "can be understood in one clear and simple concept: persistence of valid adaptations to danger into a time of safety afterward" (2002, p. 149).

PTSD does not automatically occur after trauma. So while an estimated 70% of adults in the United States have experienced a traumatic event at least once in their lives, only approximately 20% of them go on to develop PTSD, and an estimated 5% of Americans – more than 13 million people – have PTSD at any given time. Some trauma survivors have some symptoms of PTSD, but do not meet all the criteria. For example, most survivors of child abuse do not meet the full criteria for PTSD, but more than 80% are reported to have some posttraumatic symptoms.

There are four groups of symptoms, and a person must have all four to qualify for the diagnosis:

- Reexperiencing. This may occur via recurrent, involuntary, and intrusive memories; traumatic nightmares; dissociative reactions (e.g., flashbacks) anywhere on a continuum from brief episodes to complete loss of consciousness; intense or prolonged distress after exposure to traumatic reminders; or marked physiologic reactivity after exposure to trauma-related stimuli (e.g. sweating, pounding heart, or nausea).
- Avoidance. This is persistent effortful avoidance of distressing trauma-related thoughts or feelings, or trauma-related external reminders (e.g., people, places, conversations, activities, objects, or situations that remind the person of the trauma). The person may feel detached from others and emotionally numb, or lose interest in activities and life in general.
- Negative alterations in cognition and mood that began or worsened after the traumatic event. These may be an inability to recall key features of the traumatic event; persistent – and often distorted – negative beliefs and expectations about oneself or the world (e.g., "I am bad," "The world is completely dangerous"); persistent distorted blame of self or others for causing the traumatic event or for resulting consequences; persistent negative trauma-related emotions (e.g., fear, horror, anger, guilt, or shame); markedly diminished interest in (pre-trauma) significant activities; feeling alienated from others (e.g., detachment or estrangement); or persistent inability to experience positive emotions.
- Trauma-related alterations in arousal and reactivity that began or worsened after the traumatic event: irritable or aggressive behavior; self-destructive or reckless behavior; or hypervigilance (being on constant "red alert").

In recognition of the significance of complex trauma – vis-à-vis the focus on single-incident trauma that is typically connected with PTSD – The International Society for Traumatic Stress Syndrome (ISTSS) has presented additional criteria for what it terms "complex PTSD." ISTSS has noted that survivors of complex trauma may experience symptoms in the following five clusters: emotional regulation difficulties (such as impulsivity, self-destructive behaviors, or emotional constriction); disturbances in relational capacities (such as alterations in the view of oneself and of others); alterations in attention or consciousness (such as dissociation); somatic distress (such as chronic pain or other physiological symptoms); and adversely affected belief systems.

Obsessive-Compulsive and Related Disorders

Obsessive-Compulsive Disorder (OCD)

Yet another term that we throw around inaccurately in casual speech is "OCD." People tend to say, "I'm so OCD" when they are particular about certain things. In reality, OCD involves an obsession and/or compulsion that actively interfere(s) with key aspects of life, such as work, school, and personal relationships. The person spends at least one hour a day on these thoughts or behaviors; does not derive pleasure when performing the behaviors or rituals, but may feel brief relief from the anxiety the thoughts cause; and experiences significant problems in their daily life due to these thoughts or behaviors.

Obsessions are repeated thoughts, urges, or mental images that cause anxiety. Common groups include: fear of germs or contamination; unwanted or taboo thoughts involving sex, religion, and harm; aggressive thoughts towards others or self; or having things symmetrical or in a perfect order. Compulsions are repetitive behaviors that a person feels the urge to carry out in response to an obsessive thought. Common groups of compulsions include: excessive cleaning and/or handwashing; ordering and arranging things in a particular, precise way; repeatedly checking on things, such as whether the door is locked or the oven is off; and compulsive counting.

Body Dysmorphic Disorder

This involves a preoccupation with physical features that are perceived as flawed, though this is not apparent or a matter of concern to others. There is a repetitive behavioral component focused on the perceived physical anomaly, such as obsessively examining oneself in the mirror, grooming to hide or fix the perceived flaw, or seeking reassurance from others about appearance without satisfaction. The typical age of onset is 12–13, with an average onset of 16–17. Incidence in the U.S. is 2.5% in males and 2.2% in females.

Other types of obsessive-compulsive-related behaviors include hoarding, trichotillomania (chronic hair pulling), and excoriation (chronic skin pulling).

Psychotic Disorders

Psychotic disorders are severe disorders that cause abnormal thinking and perceptions. While psychosis can be a feature of a manic episode of bipolar I disorder, the most common illnesses in which psychosis is a feature are schizophrenia spectrum disorders. These are highly complex disorders, generally with what are termed "positive symptoms" such as delusions (fixed false beliefs), hallucinations (hearing voices, seeing visions), and thought disorder (as evidenced by speech that makes little sense) as well as "negative symptoms" such as withdrawal, lack of motivation, and a flat or inappropriate mood. Onset is typically between 15 and 25 years of age, and the prevalence of psychosis (including schizophrenia) is reported to be a little more than 1% throughout the world.

Personality Disorders

A personality disorder is a way of thinking, feeling, and behaving that differs significantly from what is typical in a given context. In a personality disorder, one set of characteristics is overemphasized at the expense of all others, which tend to be underdeveloped. When you are interacting with someone with a personality disorder, the characteristics described in this section are ones you encounter almost all the time, not occasionally in the way you might notice some of them in most people. The pattern of experience and behavior begins by late adolescence or early adulthood, and causes distress or problems in functioning. Without treatment, the behavior and experience are inflexible and usually long-lasting. The pattern is seen in at least two of these areas: 1) thoughts about oneself and others; 2) emotional responses; 3) relating to other people; 4) behavioral control.

There are ten specific types of personality disorders, which may be divided into three groups based on the type of central characteristic:

Cluster A: Odd or Eccentric Behavior

Paranoid personality disorder: a pattern of distrust and suspiciousness in which others' motives are seen as mean or spiteful.

Schizoid personality disorder: a pattern of detachment from social relationships and a limited range of emotional expression. This is different from social anxiety disorder/social phobia, where the person wants to have social relationships but feels that they cannot.

Schizotypal personality disorder: a pattern of acute discomfort in close relationships, distortions in thinking or perception, and eccentric behavior. A person with schizotypal personality disorder may have odd beliefs or magical thinking, odd or peculiar behavior or speech, or may incorrectly attribute meanings to events. They are not overtly psychotic, but come across as "odd."

Cluster B: Dramatic, Emotional, or Erratic Behavior

Antisocial personality disorder: a pattern of disregarding or violating the rights of others. A person with antisocial personality disorder may not conform to social norms, may repeatedly lie or deceive others, or may act impulsively, usually without remorse. This is what in day-to-day speech we refer to as a "psychopath" or "sociopath."

Borderline personality disorder: a pattern of instability in personal relationships, emotional response, self-image, and impulsivity. A person with borderline personality disorder may go to great lengths to avoid abandonment (real or perceived), display inappropriate intense anger, or display emotions towards others that tend to swing between extremes.

Histrionic personality disorder: a pattern of excessive emotion and attention-seeking via sexuality. A person with histrionic personality disorder may consistently use physical appearance to draw attention, and may show rapidly shifting or exaggerated emotions.

Narcissistic personality disorder: a pattern of need for admiration and lack of empathy for others. A person with narcissistic personality disorder tends to have a grandiose sense of self-importance and entitlement, and take advantage of others or lack empathy.

Cluster C: Anxious or Fearful Behavior

Avoidant personality disorder: a pattern of social inhibition, feelings of inadequacy, and extreme sensitivity to criticism. A person with avoidant personality disorder may be unwilling to get involved with people unless he/she is certain of being liked, and avoids intimacy for fear of rejection (as opposed to the person with social anxiety disorder who avoids social interactions for fear of judgment).

Dependent personality disorder: a pattern of needing to be taken care of and submissive/clingy behavior. A person with dependent personality disorder may have difficulty making daily decisions without reassurance from others or may feel uncomfortable or helpless when alone because of fear of inability to take care of himself/herself.

Obsessive-compulsive personality disorder: a pattern of preoccupation with perfectionism and control. A person with obsessive-compulsive personality disorder may be preoccupied with details or schedules, may work excessively to the exclusion of leisure or friendships, or may be inflexible in morality and values. This person can have a hard time letting things go figuratively (making them judgmental) or literally (leading to hoarding).

A Couple of Other Points on Diagnosis

As you saw from the descriptions in the previous section, a person needs to meet relatively specific criteria in order to qualify for a diagnosis. What if she meets some, but not all, of the criteria? In that case, she may qualify for an "other" category within the general diagnosis. For example, someone who does not meet the full criteria for any of the anxiety disorders given earlier may receive a diagnosis of "other specified anxiety disorder" or "unspecified anxiety disorder."

Sometimes, mood or anxiety symptoms show up in response to a stressful life event, but the person does not meet the criteria for a specific anxiety or mood disorder. In that case, he may qualify for a diagnosis of adjustment disorder. Adjustment disorder may be with depressed mood, with anxiety, with depressed mood and anxiety, with disturbance of conduct, or with mixed disturbance of emotions and conduct.

Dual Diagnosis

As mentioned previously, dual diagnosis refers to the co-occurrence of a mental health diagnosis with an addiction. According to a 2014 National Survey on Drug Use and Health, 7.9 million people in the U.S. experience a mental disorder and substance use disorder simultaneously (Center for Behavioral Health Statistics and Quality, 2015). Either disorder can develop first. People experiencing a mental health condition may turn to alcohol or other drugs as a form of self-medication to mitigate the mental health symptoms they are experiencing. But also, research shows that alcohol and other drugs may worsen the symptoms of mental illnesses during both intoxication and withdrawal. Studies have suggested that problems with alcohol abuse may lead to an increased risk of depression, and also that stopping drinking – even at moderate levels – may lead to health problems, including depression and reduced neurogenesis (capacity of the brain to produce new neurons) (Nordqvist, 2017).

The Three-Pronged Model Revisited

If you have been unfamiliar with emotional health diagnoses until now, you may be feeling a little inundated with all the new information we just discussed. Do remember that it is there for your referral, and that you can return to it in stages based on your needs. In addition, the Three-Pronged Model we introduced in Chapter 1 provides an easy framework for understanding and working with the general categories of these emotional imbalances.

It is helpful to see that in any imbalance – whether it fits into a diagnosis category or not – there is chronic dysregulation in the body. Because adaptation to trauma is physiological/ biological as well as psychological/ emotional, cognitive reframing alone (shifting one's mind to think about things differently) does not eradicate the trauma response. When triggered by trauma symptoms, a person's frontal lobe – responsible for reasoning – shuts down, and the limbic system, which is responsible for emotions, takes over. That is why it can be impossible to "think positive" when flooded by trauma symptoms. Furthermore, research has shown that trauma creates damage to Broca's area in the brain, which is responsible for speech production. This means that it is difficult to access language to talk about the true core of trauma (van der Kolk, 2017).

Yoga allows trauma processing not only via *manomaya kosha* (the mental body) but also by means of *annamaya kosha* in the form of *asana*, and/or *pranamaya kosha* through breathwork. But, just as a general population class may not be suitable for someone with a severe physical injury, a person who has undergone trauma typically needs a yoga experience that is more tailor-made. Let us revisit the Three-Pronged Model to see how we would use it in light of this information.

Grounding

We start every practice with grounding, and remain there as long as is necessary. It is far better to play it safe and spend too long on grounding than to move forward too quickly (see Chapter 5 on how to evaluate this). In general, we can never ground too much. Just think of yourself during your busy day and throughout your hectic life. As you move through your day in the distraction of *viksipta* that most of us inhabit at least from time to time, wouldn't you appreciate having an opportunity to become more grounded?

There are also two groups of imbalances that necessitate working with grounding even in the long term. The first is those where there is a potential or actual break with reality. The most obvious context in which this happens is psychosis. So, for bipolar disorders with psychotic features and schizophrenia, our work will only be grounding, regardless of the type of medication that the client is taking. Another context where there is a break with reality is in trauma disorders such as acute stress disorder and PTSD. The brain of a person with posttraumatic stress responds as if it were still experiencing the traumatic event, so building concentration on the present is crucial. Similarly, grounding is the priority in personality disorders, where emotional dysregulation is frequent.

Grounding is also important when there are two sets of symptoms that pull a person in different directions. For example, we mentioned that symptoms of anxiety and depression coexist in 60% of cases. As psychologist Bo Forbes points out,

> the mind and body wire *mixtures* of anxiety and depression, rather than just one or the other, into us ... The mind, for example, can be highly anxious (with rapid and worried thoughts) while at the same time, the body can be slowed-down and lethargic. On the other hand, the body can be physically agitated and much too energized, while the mind functions slowly and with difficulty.

(2011, p 21)

Similarly, for clients with bipolar disorder, research has shown that yoga can trigger mania in clients in a bipolar disorder depressive episode, and a depressive episode in clients experiencing mania (Uebelacker, Weinstock, & Kraines, 2014). Grounding is therefore imperative.

Brahmana

In cases where a client presents with symptoms associated with lethargy (*mudha*), after suitable grounding, a *brahmana* practice is advised. Symptoms of lethargy are mainly associated with depressive disorders that have melancholic (rather than anxious) features. Working with a *brahmana* practice without first grounding the client can result in a sense of instability, vulnerability, and lack of safety. But once grounding has been established, we can focus on meeting the client somewhere close to his energy level (we will discuss this more in Chapter 6), and work gradually to raise his energy.

Langhana

In instances when a client presents with symptoms associated with agitation and anxiety (*ksipta*), after suitable grounding, a *langhana* practice is advised. Symptoms of agitation are mainly associated with anxiety disorders and obsessive-compulsive-related disorders. Again, working with a *langhana* practice without first grounding the client can result in a sense of instability, vulnerability, and lack of safety. But once grounding has been established, we can focus on meeting the client somewhere close to her energy level (we will discuss this more in Chapter 7), and work gradually to calm her energy.

Yoga as an approach to treatment for trauma differs radically from current standards of care. Instead of a focus on symptom reduction by addressing negative thought patterns, troubling memories, or feared stimuli, yoga assists survivors in using the body and breath to become aware of felt experiences and to take care of themselves in the present moment, whatever arises. That means that yoga practices can serve both as preventive care in maintaining emotional balance as well as an in-the-moment go-to when symptoms arise. In the next chapter, our final one on background, we will look at some of the research on how yoga affects emotional health.

References

American Psychiatric Association. (2013). *Diagnostic and statistical manual of mental disorders* (5th ed.). Washington, DC: American Psychiatric Publishing.

Brisbon, N. M., & Lowery, G. A. (2011). Mindfulness and levels of stress: A comparison of beginner and advanced hatha yoga practitioners. *Journal of Religion and Health, 50*(4), 931–941. doi: 10.1007/s10943-009-9305-3

Broad, W. J. (2012). *The science of yoga: The risks and the rewards.* New York, NY: Simon & Schuster.

Carrera, J. (2005). *Inside the Yoga Sutras: A comprehensive sourcebook for the study & practice of Patanjali's Yoga Sutras.* Buckingham, VA: Integral Yoga Publications.

Center for Behavioral Health Statistics and Quality. (2015). Behavioral health trends in the United States: Results from the 2014 National Survey on Drug

Use and Health (HHS Publication No. SMA 15–4927, NSDUH Series H-50). Retrieved April 8, 2018 from www.samhsa.gov/data/

Cope, S. (2004). Introduction. In A. Weintraub (Ed.), *Yoga for depression: A compassionate guide to relieve suffering through yoga* (pp. xi–xiv). New York, NY: Harmony Books.

Coward, H. (2002). *Yoga and psychology: Language, memory, and mysticism.* Albany, NY: SUNY Press.

Dalal, A. S. (1991). *Psychology, mental health & yoga.* Twin Lakes, WI: Lotus Press.

Douglass, L. (2011). Thinking through the body: The conceptualization of yoga as therapy for individuals with eating disorders. *Eating Disorders, 19*(1), 83–96. doi: 10.1080/10640266.2011.533607

Evans, G. W., & Kim, P. (2013). Childhood poverty, chronic stress, self-regulation, and coping. *Child Development Perspectives, 7*(1), 43–48. doi:10.1111/cdep.12013

Follette, V., Palm, K., & Pearson, A. (2006). Mindfulness and trauma: Implications for treatment. *Journal of Rational-Emotive & Cognitive Behavior Therapy, 24*(1), 45–61. doi: 10.1007/s10942-006-0025-2

Forbes, B. (2011). *Yoga for emotional balance: Simple practices to help relieve anxiety and depression.* Boulder, CO: Shambhala Publications.

Ford, J. D., & Courtois, C. A. (2009). Defining and understanding complex trauma and complex traumatic stress disorders. In C. A. Courtois & J. D. Ford (Eds.), *Treating complex traumatic stress disorders: An evidence-based guide* (pp. 13–30). New York, NY: Guilford Press.

Hair, N. L., Hanson, J. L. Wolfe, B. L., & Pollak, S. D. (2015). Association of child poverty, brain development, and academic achievement. *JAMA Pediatrics, 169*(9), 822–829. doi:10.1001/jamapediatrics.2015.1475

Kessler, R. C., Petukhova, M., Sampson, N. A., Zaslavsky, A. M., & Wittchen, H.U. (2012). Twelve-month and lifetime prevalence and lifetime morbid risk of anxiety and mood disorders in the United States. *International Journal of Methods in Psychiatric Research, 21*(3), 169–184. doi: 10.1002/mpr.1359

Kessler, R. C., Soukup, J., Davis, R. B., Foster, D. F., Wilkey, S. A., Van Rompay, M. I., & Eisenberg, D. M. (2001). The use of complementary and alternative therapies to treat anxiety and depression in the United States. *American Journal of Psychiatry, 158*(2), 289–294. doi: 10.1176/appi.ajp.158.2.289

Kinser, P. A., Bourgignon, C., Whaley, D., Hauenstein, E., & Taylor, A. G. (2013). Feasibility, acceptability, and effects of gentle hatha yoga for women with major depression: Findings from a randomized controlled mixed-methods study. *Archives of Psychiatric Nursing, 27*(3), 137–147. doi: 10.1016/j.apnu.2013.01.003

Levine, M. (2009). *The positive psychology of Buddhism and yoga: Paths to a mature happiness.* New York & London: Routledge.

Lilly, M., & Hedlund, J. (2010). Yoga therapy in practice: Healing childhood sexual abuse with yoga. *International Journal of Yoga Therapy, 20,* 120–130. Retrieved from https://yogafordepression.com/wp-content/uploads/healing-childhood-sexual-abuse-with-yoga-lilly-and-hedlund.pdf

Lowen, A. (1972). *Depression and the body: The biological basis of faith and reality.* New York, NY: Coward, McCann & Geoghegan.

Maslow, A. (1971). *Farther reaches of human nature.* New York, NY: Arkana/Penguin Books.

MediLexicon (n. d.). Mental health. Retrieved April 8, 2018 from www.medilexicon.com/dictionary/39451

Nordqvist, C. (2017, August 24). What is mental health? *Medical News Today*. Healthline Media UK Ltd., Brighton, UK. Retrieved April 8, 2018 from www.medicalnewstoday.com/articles/154543.php

Rhodes, A. (2015). Claiming peaceful embodiment through yoga in the aftermath of trauma. *Complementary Therapies in Clinical Practice, 21*(4), 247–256. doi: 10.1016/j.ctcp.2015.09.004

Shay, J. (2002). *Odysseus in America: Combat trauma and the trials of homecoming*. New York, NY: Scribner.

Soni A. (2009, July). The five most costly conditions, 1996 and 2006: Estimates for the U.S. civilian noninstitutionalized population. Statistical Brief #248. Rockville, MD: Agency for Healthcare Research and Quality. Retrieved from www.meps.ahrq.gov/mepsweb/data_files/publications/st248/stat248.pdf

Telles, S., Singh, N., & Balkrishna, A. (2012). Managing mental health disorders resulting from trauma through yoga: A review. *Depression Research and Treatment*. Article ID 401513, 9 pages. doi:10.1155/2012/401513

Tucci, V., & Moukaddam, N. (2017). We are the hollow men: The worldwide epidemic of mental illness, psychiatric and behavioral emergencies, and its impact on patients and providers. *Journal of Emergencies, Trauma, and Shock, 10*(1), 4–6. doi:10.4103/0974-2700.199517

Uebelacker, L., Weinstock, L. M., & Kraines, M. A. (2014). Self-reported benefits and risks of yoga in individuals with bipolar disorder. *Journal of Psychiatric Practice, 20*(5), 345–352.

van der Kolk, B. A. (2017, October 23). *Trauma Foundations, Part I*. Lecture presented at 2017–2018 Certificate Program in Traumatic Stress Studies at the Trauma Center in Brookline, MA.

Weintraub, A. (2004) *Yoga for depression: A compassionate guide to relieve suffering through yoga*. New York, NY: Harmony Books.

Weintraub, A. (2015). Yoga and mental health: The crumbling wall. In E. G. Horovitz & S. Elgelid (Eds.), *Yoga and mental health: Theory and practice* (pp. 161–171). New York & London: Routledge.

World Health Organization (2012, October 10). Depression: A global crisis. Retrieved April 8, 2018 from www.who.int/mental_health/management/depression/wfmh_paper_depression_wmhd_2012.pdf

World Health Organization (2018a, March). Mental health: Strengthening our response. Retrieved April 8, 2018, from www.who.int/mediacentre/factsheets/fs220/en/

World Health Organization (2018b, March 22). Depression. Retrieved June 21, 2018 from www.who.int/news-room/fact-sheets/detail/depression

World Health Organization (n. d.). Suicide data. Retrieved April 8, 2018 from www.who.int/mental_health/prevention/suicide/suicideprevent/en/

3 How Yoga Affects Mental/ Emotional Health

In an article published in 2013, neuroscientist Stephanie Shorter estimated that yoga research in peer-reviewed publications had increased ten-fold over the previous couple of decades. At the time of her writing, she counted 74 studies that had been published just that year. When it comes to emotional health specifically, scores of articles to date have been authored on the effect of yoga on well-being. The subset focusing on mental health imbalances is significantly smaller, but nonetheless has burgeoned considerably.

Preliminary Research

One of the earliest research articles on the benefit of yoga for shifting emotional imbalance was a 1974 study of nine patients diagnosed as "anxiety neurotic" (what would now be described as generalized anxiety disorder) who practiced yoga meditation for 20 minutes, twice a day (Girodo, 1974). After approximately four months of practice, the five patients with a shorter history of illness (an average of 14.2 months) improved significantly, while the four who had a longer history (an average of 44.2 months) did not show an appreciable decline in anxiety symptoms. However, when those four were guided in relaxation while imagining the worst thing that could happen in a variety of anxiety-provoking situations, such as at work, a party, or a hockey game, their anxiety symptoms decreased. In other words, their symptoms diminished when exposed to another aspect of a yoga practice: relaxation.

This study, despite methodological laxities such as small sample size and lack of a control group, provides kernels of evidence-based research on the effectiveness of yoga on emotional imbalance. In subsequent years, research trials have similarly utilized qualitative self-report and/ or quantitative psychosocial measures – such as the Beck Depression and Anxiety Inventories or the Profile of Mood States – to assess the impact of yoga in reducing a number of emotional imbalance symptoms. Over the past two decades, a new kind of research has emerged: one that makes use of biomarker measurements such as biochemical analysis, brain scans, and physiological measurements to measure these effects.

It is, of course, impossible to discuss all – or even a significant portion of – the research on yoga and emotional health, but we can trace its main trajectories. Among the earliest relevant work that we encounter is regarding two elements encompassed in yoga: physical and meditative activity.

Physical Activity

From the mid-1980s there has been increased exploration into the role of exercise in improving emotional well-being. This body of research has suggested that moderate regular exercise should be considered as a viable means of treating depression and anxiety and improving mental well-being in the general public (Bennett, Weintraub, & Khalsa, 2008; Fox, 1999; Ströhle, 2009). This has led to the common recommendation that treatment prescriptions for emotional health include an exercise component when feasible.

Meditative Activity

The other yoga-related area in which there has been a good amount of research is meditation. Among the earliest scientists to work on the effect of meditation on emotional health was Douglas Burns, an American psychiatrist who lived in Thailand for over a decade in the 1970s. Burns became interested in personality changes taking place over a period of years in Europeans and Americans who had ordained as monks and practiced *Vipassana* meditation. Burns had noticed that of his subjects, some appeared to have "done pretty well," meaning that "the fellow is less depressed, more self-confident … He's happier, understands himself better, has better control over himself" (Burns & Ohayv, 1980, p. 15). Burns expected to have completed by late 1977 his final test results with 30 subjects and a large control group, but he disappeared mysteriously before doing so.

Psychologists have utilized meditation in clinical settings because it offers the benefits of relieving depression, reducing stress and anxiety, aiding in coping with chronic pain, decreasing sleep disturbance, and improving several domains of cognition. What is interesting is that meditation does not necessarily lower symptoms, but rather, enables noticing them non-reactively. In some ways similarly to the witness consciousness we discussed in Chapter 1, meditation enables practitioners to become detached observers of their own mental activity, so they may identify its habits and distortions (Follette et al., 2006; Kabat-Zinn, 2003).

In one study (Lin, Chang, Zemon, & Milarsky, 2008) investigating the effects of meditation on musical performance anxiety and performance quality, 19 participants from music conservatories were randomly assigned to either an eight-week meditation group or a wait-list control group. Participants in the experimental group met for 75 minutes, once a week, for eight weeks, to receive group meditation training, and were also expected to practice meditation on their own for approximately 20 minutes daily. When it came time for the performance, while participants practicing meditation reported being as anxious as participants in the control group, their performances were better. They accepted the physical manifestations of anxiety without taking on the adverse brain chatter. For example, one participant in the meditation group described her performance as "the most relaxed I had been during a solo performance in a long time, despite the fact that I was still incredibly nervous." She noted that she was aware of her feelings during the moment, "without getting caught up in the emotional reactions to the situation" (p. 150). The control group, on the other hand, demonstrated a decrease in performance quality with increases in performance anxiety, having thoughts along the lines of "my heartbeat is going fast; I am afraid that I will mess everything up" (pp. 148–149).

This awareness of the moment is what is referred to as mindfulness. Research on mindfulness has steadily increased in the last four decades, especially with the work of Jon Kabat-Zinn, creator of the Center for Mindfulness in Medicine, Health Care, and Society at the University of Massachusetts Medical School. In 1979, Kabat-Zinn developed Mindfulness Based Stress Reduction (MBSR), a combination of mindfulness meditation, body awareness, and yoga that cultivates intentionally non-reactive moment-to-moment awareness. MBSR has been shown to be effective in reducing depression, psychological distress, anxiety, sleep, and somatic complaints, and more recently neuroscience has associated it with functional brain changes, and emotional and attention improvements (Kimbrough, Magyari, Langenberg, Chesney, & Berman, 2010).

Mindfulness has been called "the heart" of Buddhist meditation. But, Kabat-Zinn has noted, mindfulness is also universal – there is nothing particularly Buddhist about it. For example, counting one's breath and noticing sounds are mindfulness exercises. In mindfulness, thoughts and feelings are not suppressed or analyzed for content, but rather, are observed non-judgmentally as they occur, moment by moment (Baer, Fischer, & Huss, 2005; Follette et al., 2006; Kabat-Zinn, 2003; Lin et al., 2008; Reibel, Greeson, Brainard, & Rosenzwig, 2001). Through openness and curiosity, one's relationship with negative thoughts is altered. Mindfulness can be considered a metacognitive skill – cognition about one's cognition (Lin et al., 2008).

Combining the Physical and the Meditative

If physical and meditative activity have each been shown to have a positive effect on mental health, we can envision that a practice encompassing the two would be even more impactful. Mental and physical (MAP) training, a novel clinical intervention that combines mental training through meditation and physical training via aerobic exercise, has been indicated to increase neurogenesis (the capacity of the brain to produce new neurons). In one study (Alderman, Olson, Brush, & Shors, 2016), 22 participants with symptoms of major depressive disorder (MDD) and 30 healthy individuals completed an eight-week intervention, consisting of two sessions per week of 30 minutes of meditation and 30 minutes of moderate-intensity aerobic exercise. Following the intervention, all participants reported significantly fewer symptoms of depression; those with MDD also reported fewer ruminative thoughts, a feature of anxious depression.

While the details of MAP may be novel, the combination of the physical and the meditative is precisely what is captured in yoga. Ross and Thomas (2010) report in their review of 12 existing studies that in healthy individuals, yoga has been shown to be as effective as or superior to exercise on nearly every outcome measured. The results of a study by Field, Diego, and Hernandez-Reif (2010) demonstrate that a yoga/Tai chi session both raised heart rate, as would be expected for moderate-intensity exercise, and increased relaxation, including lowering anxiety and augmenting the EEG theta activity associated with deep meditation. In one study (Netz & Lidor, 2003) assessing state anxiety, depressive mood, and subjective well-being among 147 female teachers prior to and following a single session of one of four exercise modes – yoga, Feldenkrais (awareness through movement), aerobic dance, and swimming – with a computer class serving as a control, results showed mood improvement following Feldenkrais, swimming, and yoga, but not following aerobic dance or the control computer lessons. The results suggest that repetitive, low-exertion rhythmical movements – which may include also swimming's meditative stroke regulation and movement against resistance – may be more powerful in mood enhancement than high-intensity movements.

Research Challenges

Certainly, we can see the promise of research results regarding the impact of yoga on emotional health. However, our eagerness for these outcomes should not lead us to have blinders on. Research on yoga is in many ways in its infancy, and as a result, only a fraction of studies have employed methodological rigor. This is in part due to cost: publishing a study with a 12-week protocol that uses both questionnaires and biomedical markers can easily cost at least $200,000 (Shorter, 2013).

The following are methodological challenges that we come across in some of the research:

Small Sample Size

Many of the studies involve a limited number of participants, which restricts quantitative analysis and generalizability. Meta-analytic reviews (articles summarizing previous research) are likewise based on a small number of studies (Kinser, Bourgignon, Whaley, Hauenstein, & Taylor, 2013; Woolery, Myers, Sternlieb, & Zeltzer, 2004).

The issue of sample size is further affected by attrition, whereby in some studies participation goes down by one third or even one half at each stage. This means that if participants dropped out because the yoga program did not work for them, there is no way to factor that into the results.

Lack of Sample Diversity

Most research on yoga is focused on what are termed "WEIRD" subjects (Western, educated, and from industrialized, rich, and democratic countries). In the United States, yoga practitioners tend to be wealthy, college-educated females of European descent with an average age of 39, and therefore, by extension, therapeutic yoga research subjects also skew in that direction (Rhodes, 2015; Shorter, 2013). In a review of research articles on depression, Karen Pilkington and her colleagues noted that "none of the participants in the yoga interventions in any study were over 50 years of age" (Pilkington, Kirkwood, Rampes, & Richardson, 2005, p. 21). And they were not only young, but also relatively fit, raising questions about the generalizability of the benefits of yoga for less healthy participants (Pilkington et al., 2005; Telles, Singh, & Balkrishna, 2012). In their research at a British university on the effectiveness of yoga for the improvement of well-being and resilience to stress in the workplace, Hartfiel, Havenland, Khalsa, Clarke, and Krayer (2011) reported that men comprised 10% of the study participants in contrast to 42% of the staff employed.

The issue of lack of diversity in age and gender is not specific to a Western context, either. In a study on the effects of yoga on depression in older adults in Taiwan, for instance, there was an underrepresentation of men aged 75 and over. The authors explain that this "may be due to a lower number of men available for the intervention or to lower acceptability of the intervention to men." Similarly, they point out that the "study sample was comprised of healthy older adults who had less than one chronic illness, on average, which may be very different from the elderly population in general" (Chen at al., 2009, p. 162).

Volunteer Bias

When it comes to recruitment, it is more likely that studies will attract subjects who are curious about practicing yoga (Shorter, 2013), and "it is well known that patient belief and expectancy can influence medical outcomes" (Reibel et al., 2001, p. 191). Volunteer bias can occur even in studies that do not name the intervention at the time of recruitment, since there is still a bias towards subjects whose socioeconomic status and symptom level place them in a position to enact changes for self-care and mental wellness (cf. Kinser et al., 2013).

Focus on Self-Report

While there has been an increase in studies relying on biomarkers, most studies still use self-report. In addition to the challenge that self-report can be colored by expectations and other agendas, in some studies the issue is compounded by the fact that questionnaires are not anonymous and may even be administered by a non-neutral party such as the instructor of the yoga class herself (e.g. Bennett et al., 2008).

Variability in Intervention

Studies range in the type of intervention used. Occasionally, the program studied involves additional interventions such as art projects or mindful eating (cf. Lilly & Hedlund, 2010). But even when the intervention is only a yoga class, it typically comprises several components such as breath, posture, sound, and meditation, making it difficult to determine whether the mood-enhancing effects of yoga are general or specific to certain components, approaches, or teachers. Of course, yoga is a complete intervention, and if different aspects are delivered separately, such a reductionist approach may result in loss of efficacy or effectiveness. Having said that, it would still be worthwhile to tease out specific results.

Confounding Factors

Studies can include other factors that may muddy the waters when it comes to interpreting results. For example, the simple act of bringing participants together in a group and therefore strengthening their social environment may be an intervention in itself, regardless of the activity in which the group then partakes (cf. Kinser et al., 2013).

Short Duration of Treatment

Studies often assess the effects of a yoga intervention over a select number of weeks, with potential follow-up months later. However, there is very little data on how the practice of yoga affects emotional health for any time over six months, and definitely not over the span of years.

No Research on Experienced Yogis

Related to this issue is that most studies recruit new yoga practitioners, and few focus on experienced ones. In one of the few comparing practitioners with less than five years of practice to those with over five years of practice, researchers Nicholas M. Brisbon and Glenn A. Lowery (2011) point out that even this approach, which does take a number of years of practice into account, does not offer any information regarding regularity of practice. "Two individuals who have practiced Hatha Yoga for the same number of years," they elucidate, "may differ in measures of stress and mindfulness if the consistency of practice differs between both individuals" (p. 939).

Control Group Challenges

Several studies lack a control group, leading to difficulties in assessing how much of the reported symptom reduction could be attributed to a placebo effect or the natural waxing and waning of symptoms over time. In others, the control group receives no intervention at all, ultimately leading to bias from participants based on whether they received an intervention or not, regardless of what that intervention was. Studies of this nature simply demonstrate that yoga (or whatever component of it is being studied) is more effective than nothing at all, not that it is more effective than other interventions. Finally, in some studies the wait-list is the control group, adding the factor of the possible effects of anticipation and expectation.

While some of these methodological challenges can be significant, by no means should they be used to dismiss the results of dozens of studies on the role of yoga in emotional health. First, a significant portion of studies have been designed in a more methodologically rigorous manner, and meta-analyses typically focus on the results of such randomized, controlled studies, even if there are fewer of them (cf. Meyer et al., 2012; Pilkington, Kirkwood, Rampes, & Richardson, 2005). Second, data from these more robust studies generally, in fact, echoes results from methodologically weaker studies (cf. Grossman, Niemann, Schmidt, & Walach, 2004; Kirkwood, Rampes, Tuffrey, Richardson, & Pilkington, 2005).

Finally, more rigorous researchers have been mindful of addressing some of the shortcomings delineated. For example, in one study of 27 women with MDD, participants were divided into a yoga group and a control group who engaged in a series of 75-minute health education sessions. Participants in both groups reported a sense of decreased depression over the course of the study, pointing to the possibility that it was the experience of coming together as a group that was effective. However, while participants in the control group suggested that they felt less depressed because they had started to care for themselves and had benefited from talking with others in the group, participants in the yoga group specifically highlighted "how connectedness occurred *transcendent* of dialogue" (Kinser et al., 2013, p. 145).

Well-Being in the General Population

There has been a significant amount of research confirming what hundreds of yoga class attendees will attest to anecdotally: yoga enhances emotional well-being in relatively healthy participants. In the abovementioned study on employees at a British university, for example (Hartfiel et al., 2011), 48 participants were randomized into either a yoga or a wait-list control group. For six weeks, the yoga group participated in a weekly hour-long class that consisted of postures, directed breathing, and relaxation techniques such as affirmation and visualization. After the six weeks, in comparison to the wait-list control group, the yoga participants reported marked improvements in feelings of clear-mindedness, composure, energy, and elation. In addition, they reported increased life purpose and satisfaction, and greater self-confidence during stressful situations.

In a study with another general population group (Varambally et al., 2013), primary caregivers (ranging in age between 18 and 60) of patients diagnosed with schizophrenia, schizoaffective disorder (a disorder marked by a combination of psychotic and mood features), and bipolar disorder with psychosis were randomized to a yoga group or a control group. Members of the yoga group were expected to attend three sessions a week for four weeks; yoga practices incorporated two direct relaxation techniques and a series of *asanas* focusing on backbends, usually used to bring about shifts in depression symptoms. After three months, the yoga group reported significant change in terms of reduction of burden and improvement in quality of life.

Emotional Imbalance

While results demonstrating the impact of yoga on general emotional health are important, the more noteworthy for our purposes are those regarding its effect on more significant imbalance. In meta-analyses on its role as a complementary treatment for psychiatric disorders, yoga has been found to be a valuable additional therapy in treating and regulating depression, anxiety, and posttraumatic stress disorder (PTSD) (Cabral, Meyer, & Ames, 2011; Kirkwood et al., 2005; Telles et al., 2012; Uebelacker, Weinstock, & Kraines, 2014; Varambally et al., 2013). Since we cannot possibly examine all the studies that have emerged discussing this, we will start here with three that cover a broad range of participants.

In one meta-analysis (da Silva, Ravindran, & Ravindran, 2009), yoga showed benefit alone or in conjunction with medication in 16 studies on mild to moderate depression, five on dysthymia (now called persistent depressive disorder), eight on anxiety, and two on obsessive-compulsive disorder (OCD). When it came to PTSD, yoga turned out to be an effective augmentation to antidepressants in four studies with Vietnam veterans, some of whom also had MDD. Yoga was also found to benefit depression and/or anxiety associated with ovarian cancer, AIDS, gastrointestinal disorders, and cardiovascular and thyroid disorders.

Another review of articles (Meyer et al., 2012) surveyed the results of 13 studies that tested the benefits of yoga in patients diagnosed with major depression, schizophrenia, PTSD, and bipolar disorder; anxiety was considered a component of the other disorders. Ten of these found significant improvement in the yoga group alone on one or more outcome measures. More specifically, the results of seven of nine studies on major depression suggested that yoga may be effective in its treatment as an adjunct intervention or even when used alone.

Finally, in a study on the effects of yoga on mood in psychiatric inpatients (Lavey et al., 2005), 113 participants took part in yoga classes that consisted of stretching and strengthening exercises, breathing, and attention to physical sensation. The group comprised 43 individuals with a mood disorder diagnosis (including bipolar disorder, major depression, or dysthymic disorder), 36 with a psychotic disorder diagnosis (including schizophrenia), nine with a borderline personality disorder diagnosis, five with an adjustment disorder diagnosis, and 20 with other diagnoses. Regardless of gender or diagnosis, participants reported significant improvements in five areas: tension-anxiety, depression-dejection, anger-hostility, fatigue-inertia, and confusion-bewilderment.

Having obtained somewhat of a general overview from these studies, let us now look into research into specific imbalances. Again, it would be impossible to cover even a significant portion of the research available, so I have selected studies with an eye to including some diversity in subject profile and location, as well as nature of intervention. At this point in time, most studies on the effects of yoga are regarding the two most commonly occurring emotional imbalances: anxiety and depression.

Anxiety

In this section, we will look specifically at four studies that provide insight into some less frequently examined aspects: one study has one-year follow-up data, two take place outside a Western context, and one includes advanced practitioners.

The first of these (Khalsa, Shorter, Cope, Wyshak, & Sklar, 2009; cf. also Khalsa & Cope, 2006 and Butzer, Ahmed, & Khalsa, 2016) focuses on performance anxiety. A group of musicians enrolled in a two-month summer fellowship program at the Tanglewood Music Center in Lenox, Massachusetts, were invited to participate in a regular yoga and meditation program at the nearby Kripalu Center for Yoga and Health. Three groups of 15 participants each were formed: a yoga lifestyle intervention group, a group practicing yoga and meditation only, and a control group who did not participate in any activities. Both yoga groups attended three Kripalu yoga or meditation classes each week, and the yoga lifestyle group also took part in weekly group practice and discussion sessions. All participants completed self-report questionnaires before and after their programs; then, in one of the few relatively long-term studies available, some participants completed a one-year follow-up assessment using the same questionnaires.

Both yoga groups showed a trend towards lowered music performance anxiety and significantly less general anxiety/tension, depression, and anger at the end of their programs, while the control group did not. Interestingly, results were similar in the two yoga groups, suggesting that the yoga and meditation techniques themselves were what was leading to the decrease in symptoms, rather than the other components of the lifestyle program such as the discussion sessions. Some of the most positive feedback, however, came in the follow-up assessment, when a number of participants reported achieving "life-changing clarity," which they attributed to the yoga practice.

The second of the studies we will explore here (Javnbakht, Hejazi Kenari, & Ghasemi, 2009) investigates the effects of yoga on depression and anxiety in women in Iran. In this study, 34 women participated in twice-weekly 90-minute yoga classes for two months, while 31 were assigned to a waiting list. Both groups were evaluated again after the two-month study period, when the women who participated in the yoga classes showed a significant decrease in both state anxiety and trait anxiety compared with at the start of the study and with the control group.

The third study (Jadhav & Havalappanavar, 2009) also examines the effect of yoga on state and trait anxiety, this time in 50 first-year students enrolled in a naturopathy and yogic sciences course at an Indian university. These students took the Spielberger State-Trait Anxiety Inventory and the Nagpal & Sell Subjective Well-being Inventory at the beginning of the academic year, and then again one year later. Results revealed a significant decrease in both state and trait anxiety scores, and positive change in the reported subjective well-being of the students.

The final study we will look at is one of the few that compare beginner and advanced practitioners (Brisbon & Lowery, 2011). The beginner group consisted of 24 individuals with between one and five years' experience in *hatha yoga*, while the advanced group comprised 28 participants ranging in experience from 6 to 30 years. Results indicated that advanced practitioners did exhibit higher levels of mindfulness and lower levels of stress when compared with beginners. More significantly, experienced practitioners were able to use their yoga practice to achieve certain physiological and therefore emotional effects: when given six minutes to reduce their heartbeats without suggestion as to how, they were able to do so more effectively.

Depression

Evidence for the effect of yoga on depression is the most robust. Even meta-analyses such as Duan-Porter et al. (2016), which dismiss results from several studies due to a high risk for bias, found that "yoga may improve short-term depressive symptoms" (p. 282). Several studies looking at co-occurring anxiety and depression symptoms find statistically significant differences between yoga and control groups on reduction of depression scores but statistically insignificant changes on anxiety scores (de Manincor et al., 2016; Uebelacker & Broughton, 2016).

Here we will look at two meta-analyses, three studies focusing specifically on practices geared towards depression, and one study of older adults. The first meta-analysis (Cramer, Lauche, Langhorst, & Dobos, 2013) surveyed 12 trials with a total of 619 participants. Results revealed moderate evidence for short-term effects on depression of yoga compared with typical psychotherapeutic care, and limited evidence compared with relaxation and aerobic exercise (more limited evidence was found for the short-term effects on anxiety of yoga compared with relaxation). In a second meta-analysis (Mehta & Sharma, 2010) of 18 studies from seven countries — Brazil (one), Canada (one), India (six), Iran (one), Japan (one), Taiwan (one), and the United States (seven) — beneficial effects were found in 17 of them. Only the one study that we discussed earlier on Iranian women (Javnbhakt et al., 2009), which demonstrated significant effects on anxiety, found no significant impact on depression.

The first of the studies specifically focused on practices for depression (Streeter et al., 2017) assessed the effects of Iyengar yoga and coherent breathing (equal length inhales and exhales at five breaths per minute) on depressive symptoms in 30 individuals. In addition to MDD, some subjects met or almost met criteria for other disorders, whether current or in remission: 13 PTSD, four panic disorder, and one social phobia. Subjects were randomized into a high-dose group or a low-dose group; over 12 weeks, the former took three yoga classes per week, while the latter took two. The 90-minute classes consisted of approximately 60 minutes of postures emphasizing the backbends and inversions identified in the Iyengar method as useful for treating depression, approximately 10 minutes of transition that included *savasana*, and then 20 minutes of coherent breathing with even inhales and exhales. Participants had homework assignments consisting of 15 minutes of postures and 15 minutes of CD-paced coherent breathing. At the end of the 12 weeks, both groups demonstrated a significant decrease in symptoms, with no significant difference between them in symptom reduction or remission.

In an earlier study also focusing on yoga postures identified within the Iyengar tradition to alleviate depression (Woolery et al., 2004) — back bends, inversions, and vigorous standing poses — 28 young adults with mild depression at a college campus recreation center were randomly assigned to a yoga course or a wait-list control group. Subjects in the yoga group attended two one-hour Iyengar yoga classes each week for five consecutive weeks, and they were not encouraged to practice at home. This is one of a minority of studies in which results were not only gathered through self-report — via the Beck Depression Inventory, the State-Trait Anxiety Inventory, and the Profile of Mood States — but also with a biomarker: morning cortisol levels.

Subjects who participated in the yoga course reported decreased levels of negative mood and fatigue following yoga classes. They also demonstrated significant decreases in self-reported symptoms of depression and trait anxiety by the middle of the yoga course, and these were maintained at the end. Furthermore, compared with controls, there was a trend for higher morning cortisol levels in the yoga group by the end of the yoga course. Although elevated cortisol responses to stress are associated with pathophysiological consequences, higher morning cortisol levels have been associated with self-esteem, hardiness, and tenacity, and lower levels of nervousness, depression, and emotional lability.

In another study of practices tailored to alleviating depression symptoms (Bennett et al., 2008), data was gathered over the course of several trainings and retreats led by LifeForce Yoga creator Amy Weintraub. The LifeForce Yoga Program incorporates postures (*asanas*), yogic breathing exercises (*pranayama*), visualization (*bhavana*), intention (*sankalpa*), hand gestures (*mudra*), chanting (*mantra*), and meditation. At the start of the study, 51% of participants scored at or above a score of 14 on the Beck Depression Inventory, indicating symptoms of at least mild depression. After two weeks, average scores for depression decreased by approximately 50%, and there were also decreases in scores for anger, fatigue, and confusion, and an increase for vigor. Furthermore, all these markers improved slightly two months later.

One of the few studies (Chen et al., 2009) in older adults comprised 128 participants (62 experimental, 66 control) with an average age of 69.20, who were recruited from eight Taiwan senior activity centers. The experimental group participated in a 70-minute senior yoga exercise program, three times per week, for six months. The program included warm-ups, appropriate *asanas*, abdominal breathing, relaxation, and guided-imagery meditation. At the end of the six months, the yoga group reported better sleep quality, physical health perception, and mental health perception, and lower daytime dysfunction and depression states.

PTSD

Among the most significant research on the effects of yoga on PTSD has come from psychiatrist Bessel van der Kolk and his colleagues at the Trauma Center in Brookline, Massachusetts, home of Trauma Sensitive Yoga. In a pilot study (van der Kolk, 2006), 37 women with severe trauma histories who had received years of therapy without much benefit were placed at random into a yoga group or a dialectical behavioral therapy (DBT; see Chapter 2) group. While yoga significantly decreased PTSD arousal symptoms and dramatically improved subjects' relationships to their bodies (for example, participants reported now listening to their bodies' needs), eight weeks of DBT did not affect arousal levels or PTSD symptoms.

In a more extensive study that ran from 2008 to 2011 (van der Kolk et al., 2014), 64 women with chronic PTSD symptoms that had also been treatment resistant were randomly assigned to a ten-week, weekly one-hour class of either trauma-informed yoga or women's health education. At the end of the study, 16 of 31 participants (52%) in the yoga group no longer met criteria for PTSD, compared with 6 of 29 (21%) in the control group. Furthermore, while both groups exhibited significant decreases in PTSD symptoms during the first half of treatment, these improvements were maintained in the yoga group, while the control group relapsed after its initial improvement.

In a related qualitative study (West, Liang, & Spinazzola, 2017), participants reported especially changes in attitudes of gratitude and compassion, relatedness, acceptance, centeredness, and empowerment. However, when 49 of the participants completed long-term follow-up interviews 18 months after the end of the initial trial (Rhodes, Spinazzola, & van der Kolk, 2016), at that point, there were no differences in PTSD symptoms between the yoga and the health education groups. Yet, those who had *continued* their yoga practice past the trial had greater decreases in both PTSD and depression symptom severity, and a greater likelihood of the loss of PTSD diagnosis. Therefore, long-term studies are crucial in determining the efficacy of yoga, and long-term practice is key.

Price et al. (2017) built on this work by examining the effect of expanding the same trauma-informed yoga treatment from a weekly ten-week program to a 20-week one, again with a sample of women with treatment-unresponsive, chronic PTSD. In addition to attending weekly sessions, participants were asked to complete three weekly 30-minute home practices using a DVD or CD. Students began their yoga practice with 15–18 minutes of seated yoga, typically on a chair. They were then invited to practice standing, seated, prone, and reclined poses, followed by three to five minutes of stillness and silence.

Based on self-report and clinical interview data, this group of participants experienced PTSD and dissociation symptom reduction beyond that of the earlier ten-week study (van der Kolk et al., 2014). Specifically, 83% of them no longer met the criteria for PTSD one week after treatment ended, while this was the case with only 52% of women in the ten-week trial. In addition, the overall sample experienced a 51% reduction in PTSD symptoms at the one-week post-treatment assessment, while participants in the ten-week trial exhibited a 33% reduction. It is also significant that women in this study exhibited a 64% reduction in PTSD at the two-month follow-up, suggesting that they continued to improve after treatment completion, and pointing to a need for longer-term treatment for women with severe and chronic PTSD.

In a longer-term project at the Trauma Center (Rhodes, 2015), 60 women aged 18 to 58 meeting criteria for PTSD, and comprising six separate cohorts over the course of three years, were divided into three yoga groups and three control groups. The average number of stressful life experiences that each of the women had endured was eight. The yoga cohorts completed a ten-week once-a-week yoga program, while the control group attended a women's health seminar. After completing their programs, participants were given the opportunity to join the following cohort in the opposite intervention, and seven women chose to do this.

Over the course of a six-month period, 49 of the 60 original participants completed long-term follow-up interviews. Two of the participants had stopped practicing yoga, 29 had continued practicing less than once per week, and eight were practicing yoga at least once per week. Participants reported an improved connection with and sense of ownership over their bodies, emotions, and thoughts, greater focus on their experiences in the present moment, a growing sense of self-efficacy, and empowerment to transcend a life that had been ruled by trauma symptoms.

Work by other groups of researchers supports these results. For instance, another randomized clinical trial (Mitchell et al., 2014) found that women with full or subthreshold PTSD symptoms showed decreases in reexperiencing and hyperarousal after 12 sessions of Kripalu yoga. Similarly, in a study on military personnel (Johnston et al., 2015), results from 12 respondents supported that study's primary hypothesis that yoga would reduce PTSD symptoms, although it did not support the hypothesis that yoga would significantly increase mindfulness.

OCD

Studies on the effect of yoga on OCD are relatively rare. In one of the most illuminating, 12 participants at Children's Hospital San Diego practiced a kundalini yoga meditation protocol, which consisted of a number of techniques including mantra meditation as well as what researchers (Shannahoff-Khalsa et al., 1999) identified as an OCD-specific technique: breathing through only the left nostril. The remaining ten participants practiced a control regimen that was also meditative, thus enabling researchers to test the hypothesis that "meditation techniques in general may not be effective" and that "disorder-specific" techniques may be required. At three months, the OCD-specific yoga group showed a 38.4% reduction in symptoms, whereas the control meditation group showed a 13.9% reduction. Based on the original outline of the program, in which if one intervention was seen to be more successful the two groups would be merged and receive it, groups were merged for an additional year using the OCD-specific technique. At 15 months, the final group of 11 participants had improved by 71% and 62%, respectively, on their scores on two OCD-specific assessment tools.

Eating Disorders and Substance Abuse

Now that we have looked at some of the research on the effects of yoga on symptoms of depression, anxiety, PTSD, and OCD, let us turn to a sampling of studies on its influence on eating disorders and substance use. We have not discussed these topics so far in this book, but will do so in Chapter 8, exploring how to apply the Three-Pronged Model to working with them.

In the studies on trauma described earlier, we emphasized the role of yoga in building internal awareness. This is especially valuable in contexts where we have a tendency to judge the body by its external appearance rather than its internal needs, such as in the case of eating disorders. For example, Jennifer Daubenmier (2005) carried out two research projects exploring the relationship of yoga, body awareness, and body responsiveness to self-objectification and disordered eating. The first compared women with an average age of 37 who were taking yoga classes with two other groups of women: one taking aerobics classes and the other taking neither. The second study did the same for a sample of younger women: 133 undergraduate students, with an average age of 20.46.

At the end of both studies, the yoga practitioners reported less self-objectification, greater satisfaction with physical appearance, and fewer disordered eating attitudes compared with the non-yoga practitioners. For the yoga practitioners, greater yoga experience in terms of number of hours practiced per week and level of expertise was associated with less self-objectification and greater body satisfaction, respectively. In keeping with previous research on the subject, among the aerobic participants the opposite was evident: more time spent doing aerobics per week was associated with greater disordered eating attitudes.

In another study (McIver, O'Halloran, & McGartland, 2009) focusing on women aged 25–65 with a body mass index (BMI) greater than 25 and a score higher than 20 on the Binge Eating Scale, participants took part in a 12-week series of weekly 60-minute yoga classes. These typically included five minutes of *pranayama*, 45 minutes of *hatha yoga*, and ten minutes of *yoga nidra* (guided sleep meditation) with meditation instruction for eating mindfully (e.g., noting the pace of their eating and quantity consumed) but not dietary advice. For the yoga group, both reductions in self-reported binge eating and increases in self-reported physical activity were statistically significant, and these changes were accompanied by statistically significant, albeit small, reductions in BMI and hip and waist measurements. Furthermore, improvements on these measures were maintained at three-month follow-up. No significant changes occurred for the control group.

These results are in contrast to an earlier study (Mitchell, Mazzeo, Rausch, & Cooke, 2007) of 93 undergraduates that examined the effectiveness of a yoga group and a cognitive dissonance-based discussion group on disordered eating symptomatology, drive for thinness, body dissatisfaction, and alexithymia (inability to identify one's emotions). While participants in the cognitive dissonance group reported a decrease in these variables at the end of the study, the yoga group did not. The authors point out that in contrast to previous studies where participants practiced for longer, perhaps the yoga intervention in this study – six weeks, 45 minutes per week – was not enough to have a significant impact on attitudes and behaviors. In addition, although the yoga intervention used meditation, it was not specific to mind–body awareness pertaining to disordered eating.

Research results on the effects of yoga on substance use have likewise been mixed. While they suggest that yoga may serve as a promising intervention for preventing substance use via mitigating risk factors such as depression or anxiety, studies on its concrete effects on addiction are limited. For example, in one study (Marefata, Peymanzad, & Alikhajeh, 2011) on depression and anxiety levels among 50 adult male recovering addicts at a community center in Iran, participants took part in three 60-minute yoga sessions per week for five weeks. At first, the sessions included breathing exercises, meditation and relaxation; then *asanas* were added. Results in the yoga group vis-à-vis the control group indicated significant differences in levels of depression and state anxiety, and insignificant alteration in levels of trait anxiety. However, we have no data on how this might have affected subsequent use or recovery.

The most favorable results on substance use are with regard to smoking. In one study (Bock et al., 2012) of women in treatment for smoking cessation, participants were divided into a yoga therapy group and a general health and wellness program group. Participants receiving yoga had higher seven-day smoking abstinence rates than controls, and abstinence remained higher among them through the six-month follow-up. Another study (Elibero, Janse Van Rensburg, & Drobes, 2011) assigned daily smokers to a yoga intervention, an exercise intervention, or a control group. Not only did the yoga and exercise groups report a decrease in cravings compared with the control group, but also the yoga group reported a *general* decrease in cravings, while the exercise group reported lower craving in response to smoking cues in particular.

How Does Yoga Work?

We can see from the research in this chapter that while some of the evidence-based data on the role of yoga for emotional health is mixed or obtained via less rigorous methodology, there are nevertheless some promising trends. What is it about yoga that helps participants find more balance? Recent findings (Gard, Noggle, Park, & Wilson, 2014; Kinser et al., 2013; Sullivan et al., 2018; Uebelacker et al., 2014) have enabled us to advance the idea that yoga can mitigate stress responses via mechanisms that are both top-down (e.g., via neurocognitive psychological appraisal) and bottom-up (e.g., via neurophysiological autonomic changes).

Gard et al. (2014) suggest that it is the meta-awareness involved in interoception (awareness of the internal state of one's body) that facilitates integration between higher-level and lower-level brain networks. They describe how yoga can affect higher-level/top-down tasks such as intention/ motivational goal setting, attentional control, response inhibition, working memory, and cognitive reappraisal, as well as lower-level/bottom-up functions that quiet the body by improving the regulatory functioning of the autonomic nervous system in the form of parasympathetic control and increased vagal tone (see later for definitions of these phenomena). In other words, yoga can support both psychological and pharmacological therapies by providing tools for greater awareness and insight, while also improving autonomic self-regulation. In the following, I will discuss these two directions, referring to them as the psychosocial and physiological effects of yoga.

Psychosocial Effects

In Chapter 1, we mentioned that yoga practitioners in the West often refer to "yoga on the mat" and "yoga off the mat." The idea is that because yoga was conceptualized as a comprehensive system, aspects that develop during a yoga practice will generalize into other areas of life. For instance, using the body and the breath to help calm the mind during a yoga class may bring about a state change affecting the moment. But the yoga practitioner may draw on that experience to calm the mind at other times, perhaps eventually leading to a trait change.

There are three "off the mat" dimensions of growth most typically reported by yoga practitioners. These are: learning to be in the present, developing a new relationship with oneself, and developing a new relationship with others. Let us explore each and its components, with the understanding that there can be some overlap between them.

Learning to Be in the Present

GROUNDING

Hatha yoga provides an entry point for feeling the body in the present moment. If I press into my feet in a standing pose, for example, I can really feel my feet, the floor, and the contact between them, therefore shifting my mind – even for a moment – into the more neutral present and away from the woes of the past or the fears of the future.

AWARENESS OF THE BODY

As we practice yoga and begin to focus our attention on our breathing and our physical sensations, we may start to notice the connection between the emotions and the body. For example, we may become aware that anxiety about doing a pose literally throws us off balance. We then begin to experiment with changing the way we feel. Will straightening the spine or focusing on the exhalation help bring about more stability? As van der Kolk notes, "Once you start approaching your body with curiosity rather than with fear, everything shifts" (2015, p. 275).

COMMUNICATION IN THE BODY

A large part of the practice in *hatha yoga* lies in sensing just how far to move into a pose. If one does not move far enough, the sense of engagement is limited. If one moves too much, that might result in pain. Therefore, yoga practitioners learn to value their body's feedback and train in "listening" to the sensations of their bodies for guidance.

By responding to these more subtle bodily cues, practitioners start to gain insight into other sensations as well, such as those related to emotions. They notice, for example, the first signs of sadness or anger, before they spiral out of control. Rather than thinking of the body as "something that must be 'disciplined' " in some way, yoga teacher Laura Douglass emphasizes, yoga practitioners see it as "an integral part of the self that needs to be listened to, cared for, and communicated with" (2011, p. 86).

LESS PHYSICAL AND EMOTIONAL RESTRICTION

When I first started yoga, I had a hard time taking long, deep breaths. Gradually, that restriction eased. And being less physically restricted translates into not only more physical openness, but also more emotional openness. One participant in Rhodes's study on PTSD articulated, "The yoga kind of made my brain relax a little bit" (2015, p. 250). As van der Kolk (2015) notes, people who feel safe in their bodies can begin to access the thoughts and memories that previously overwhelmed them.

SITTING WITH DISCOMFORT

Sometimes the experience in the body and mind during yoga is positive, but at other times it may be uncomfortable and challenging. While that can be a deterrent, if participants can stay with that physical and perhaps also emotional discomfort, it becomes an opportunity for healing. One of Rhodes's participants explained

Because I was in the yoga class experiencing all different experiences – from nothing to something really scary and all different levels – it reminded me that I will have a lot of different experiences and that if I just wait long enough it will pass.

Another remarked, "Practicing yoga definitely has allowed me to — not only with anger, but with a lot of things — given me the ability to sit with things for longer periods of time" (2015, p. 251). As van der Kolk et al. (2014) note, "Yoga may improve the functioning of traumatized individuals by helping them to tolerate physical and sensory experiences associated with fear and helplessness and to increase emotional awareness and affect tolerance" (p. e559).

SELF-REGULATION

Being able to sit with discomfort — however briefly — is a practice in self-regulation: it means we are able to handle that discomfort without coming completely out of our window of tolerance and "losing it." If I experience physical discomfort in a pose and turn to deepening my breath to ease it, I am practicing self-regulation. At first, Gard et al. (2014) argue, self-regulation occurs top-down, as yoga practitioners tell themselves to focus on the breath and notice the transient nature of their physical sensations. However, as their practice deepens, emphasis on interoception increases, and bottom-up strategies become more present. Now, regulation of the emotion-generative regions of the brain (i.e., the limbic system) may occur without having to recruit the "higher" brain regions to tell yourself that it will be ok.

BUILDING EMOTIONAL FLEXIBILITY

Have you at a point in your life been unable to see options in a situation, only to look back later and see that you had more choices than you thought you had? That is one of the challenges that come up at times of imbalance: a narrowing where it is hard to see possibilities. Sitting with discomfort and engaging in self-regulation can lead to insight about breadth of experience. If I choose to be in an uncomfortable pose and know I can come out of it, therefore shifting the discomfort, I am developing emotional flexibility. That, then, may help me gain insight into my responses to life's internal and external stressors (cf. Douglass, 2011).

New Relationship with Oneself

These aspects of change can lead to a new relationship with oneself.

SELF-CARE

When we begin paying attention to our internal states, we start engaging in self-care. For many of the women with PTSD symptoms (Rhodes, 2015), the time spent practicing yoga was the first in their lives that they had set aside to do something aimed at feeling good. In doing so, they also felt they had more control over their lives, including positive shifts in their outlooks, behaviors, and relationships. The philosophical underpinnings of yoga, captured in *yamas* such as *ahimsa* (nonviolence) and kindness to oneself, support this further.

INSIGHT AND SHIFTING PATTERNS

One participant in Kinser et al.'s study on depression (2013) commented that learning how to be mindful of the breath and body helped her break patterns of self-judging thoughts: "I normally look at all the things I didn't get done or do perfectly ... but in the class I learned to focus and be pleased with just doing a little something for me" (p. 143). Another noted that she learned to let "thoughts go by without obsessing" (p. 143). In Rhodes's study (2015), participants reported creating new insights and new ways to experience the self and make choices for themselves. Similarly, in West et al.'s study (2017), participants became aware of what they needed to feel healthy, generating gentleness with themselves and patience with the process of change, and experiencing a quieter mind and the ability to see alternative perspectives.

NOTICING POSITIVE TRAITS AND EMOTIONS

As shifts occur towards a greater sense of self-efficacy and internal peace, practitioners in various studies reported gaining more of a number of positive psychological traits and characteristics. In one study (Ross, Bevans, Friedmann, Williams, & Thomas, 2014), the majority of participants agreed that yoga improved happiness (86.5%), energy (84.5%), sleep (68.5%), and social relationships (67%). As one participant elucidated, a yoga practice brings about a calm, serene, or blissful state, whereby practitioners become " 'better' human beings: less aggressive, more flexible, more creative – without any indoctrination or imposition of a philosophical system" (p. 74).

New Relationship with Others

The category of "social relationships" delineated earlier is the third psychosocial reason why yoga may help lead to emotional balance.

MEETING OTHERS

Yoga may provide a sense of community and decrease social isolation, especially in contexts where students attend the same class with the same teacher for several weeks, months, or even years (cf. Kinser et al., 2013; Ross et al., 2014). While that could be argued to be a benefit of any group activity, yoga participants highlight the benefit of a social interaction that transcends conversation. "Shared consciousness was there, when everyone was together," one of Kinser's participants explained. "The shared centeredness is very powerful, it makes you feel a feeling of connectedness with everything … even by breathing together" (Kinser et al., 2013, p. 143).

IMPROVING RELATIONSHIP QUALITY

Just like yoga practice was found to provide coping mechanisms for the relationship with the self, it also may do this in relationship with others. In one study (Ross et al., 2014), practitioners believed that their interpersonal relationships had improved because their attitude and perspectives had changed, making them more patient, kind, mindful, and self-aware.

TRANSCENDENT CONNECTION

Although yoga brings health and harmony to the body and mind, its effects are believed to extend beyond the individual to the family and society (Ross et al., 2014). This is encapsulated in the report of the participant earlier about the rich experience of shared consciousness that she accessed just by breathing as part of a group.

Physiological Effects

In addition to its effect on top-down learning, yoga is thought to treat symptoms of certain emotional imbalances through psychophysiological, neuroendocrine, and autonomic elements related to either its aerobic components (*asana*) and/or its breathing and meditative components (*pranayama* and *dhyana*).

Balancing the Sympathetic and Parasympathetic Nervous Systems

While the effect of yoga on emotional health has been related to shifts in neurotransmitter and hormone levels, as well as brain structure, ultimately what is most significant is its role in the modulation of the autonomic nervous system (ANS). The human body has two nervous systems: the central nervous system (CNS), which is composed of the brain and the spinal cord, and the ANS, which is a network attached to and surrounding the spinal cord. The ANS operates mostly below the level of consciousness to regulate many bodily functions such as salivation, digestion, and pupil dilation, but it shares control of two elements with the CNS: muscle tension and breathing (Levine, 2009). In other words, these last two are controlled automatically, but we can also have slight control over them, and you will notice that they coincide with the practices of *asana* and *pranayama*. In recent years the ANS has also been found to play a major role in positive social behaviors such as bonding, care-giving, social communication, and emotional expression (Gerbarg & Brown, 2015).

The ANS has three wings, two of which are the sympathetic nervous system (SNS) and the parasympathetic nervous system (PNS). The SNS is responsible for arousal, including the fight or flight response. It is called "sympathetic" because it functions with the emotions (*sympathos*). The SNS moves blood to the muscles for quick action, partly by triggering the adrenal glands to secrete adrenaline, which speeds up the heart rate and increases blood pressure. The PNS promotes self-preservation functions like digestion and wound healing, and also affects facial expression and communication (Gerbarg & Brown, 2015). It is called "parasympathetic" because it functions *against* the emotions, producing a feeling of relaxation – this is why it is sometimes referred to as the "rest-and-digest" system. Parasympathetic activation is the normal resting state of your body, brain, and mind. The cooling, steadying influence of the PNS helps you think clearly and avoid hot-headed actions that would harm you or others.

These two wings of the ANS are like a seesaw: when one goes up, the other goes down. The sympathetic acts as the body's accelerator, and the parasympathetic as its brake. "Whenever you take a deep breath," explains van der Kolk,

> you activate the SNS. The resulting burst of adrenaline speeds up your heart, which explains why many athletes take a few short, deep breaths before starting competition. Exhaling, in turn, activates the PNS, which slows down the heart ... As we breathe, we continually speed up and slow down the heart.
>
> (2015, p. 79)

If as you were reading the description of the PNS, you were thinking, "But I never feel relaxed like that," then you are capturing a major challenge of our modern society. Instead of alternating between SNS arousal and PNS equilibrium, most of us spend a good amount of time in SNS activation. As Kreher explains,

> Though the stress response was meant for emergency use only, we are increasingly living in a state of SNS arousal. Our modern sabre tooth tigers are busy schedules, media overload, financial stress, long commutes, relationship discord, health problems, violence, and social injustice to name a few.
>
> (2015, p. 174)

As stress reaches a point where it is too intense or too prolonged, the PNS may become less active and the system reverts to the SNS, continuing to speed up the heart and respiration, generating angry fight or fearful flight reactions. This state is called parasympathetic withdrawal (Gerberg & Brown, 2015, p. 65).

Living in a constant state of SNS arousal has implications beyond the emotional: "it continually shunts resources away from long-term projects – such as building a strong immune system or preserving a good mood – in favor of short-term crises. And this has lasting consequences" (Mendius & Hanson, 2009, p. 55). In Chapter 2, we saw that psychological trauma results in the activation of the SNS and suppression of the PNS. "In situations where there is no possibility of fighting or running away," this reaches extreme levels, where "the SNS may default to the lowest level of defense, the vagal brake, expressed as freezing, becoming paralyzed, playing dead, fainting, or passive behavior" (Gerberg & Brown, 2015, p. 65).

Mendius and Hanson succinctly describe the three criteria we need in order to keep the autonomic nervous system in an optimal state of balance:

- Mainly parasympathetic arousal for a baseline of ease and peacefulness
- Mild SNS activation for enthusiasm, vitality, and wholesome passions
- Occasional SNS spikes to deal with demanding situations, from a great opportunity at work to a late-night call from a teenager who needs a ride home from a party gone bad (2009, p. 60).

This is where yoga comes in. Studies suggest that its controlled breathing (especially the long exhalations) and meditative practices can result in a reduction in sympathetic and an increase in parasympathetic tone, resulting in emotional regulation (Meyer et al., 2012; Visceglia, 2015). With consistent yoga practice, it may take more physical stress or more intense emotional reactivity to induce a typical "stress response" (Gard et al., 2014). At the same time, not all practices activate the PNS; hence the ability of yoga to bring about balance, and the importance of choosing the appropriate practice for the imbalance one is addressing. For instance, while slow breathing generally increases parasympathetic activity, forceful, high-frequency breathing may induce SNS and CNS activation (Meyer et al., 2012).

Vagus Nerve/Vagal Tone

The vagus nerve is the tenth of 12 cranial nerves, and is involved in parasympathetic control of the heart, lungs, and digestive tract. Its fibers are responsible for carrying sensory information from inside the body up to the brain; in other words, it is directly related to interoception. Vagal tone refers to the activity of the vagus nerve, and is associated with greater behavioral flexibility. The vagus nerve can be irritated and misfire due to a variety of reasons, such as gastrointestinal distress, muscular imbalance, or excess alcohol. Stress, anxiety, and fatigue can also inflame it, causing it to misfire and thereby affecting SNS/PNS balance.

Research has demonstrated that calming the SNS and activating the PNS stimulates the vagus nerve, leading to more adaptive top-down and bottom-up processes such as attention regulation and affective processing (Sullivan et al., 2018). Yoga practice may facilitate high vagal tone (Streeter et al., 2012). For example, Bowman et al. (1997) observed a significant increase in vagal/parasympathetic activity in healthy elderly persons after yoga, but not after aerobic exercise. Kalyani et al. (2011) found that *mantra* in the form of chanting was helpful in stimulating the vagus nerve through its auricular branches. Via functional magnetic resonance imaging (fMRI), they demonstrated the effect of audible "OM" chanting vis-à-vis a lack of effect following the pronunciation of "sss" for the same length of time (15 seconds) while in the same supine position.

Vagus nerve stimulation leads to a variety of changes, some of which we will examine later. These include an increase in heart rate variability, an increase in levels of neurotransmitters such as dopamine, norepinephrine, and serotonin, and a decrease in levels of cortisol (Kinser et al., 2013; Meyer et al., 2012).

Heart Rate Variability (HRV) and Respiratory Sinus Arrhythmia (RSA)

Heart rate variability refers to the interval between heartbeats, and reflects the activity of the autonomic nervous system. It is different from the heart rate itself, and is continually changing, speeding up a little on the inhale (SNS activation) and slowing down on the exhale (PNS arousal) (cf. Mendius & Hanson, 2009). Negative emotions decrease HRV; for example, depression is associated with low parasympathetic tone, as measured by HRV. Respiratory sinus arrhythmia (RSA) is heart rate variability in synchrony with respiration.

The controlled breathing practices, meditation, and relaxation found in yoga have been shown to increase HRV and RSA, thereby positively affecting anxiety, panic disorder, and depression (Gard et al., 2014; Kinser et al., 2013; Meyer et al., 2012). For example, Streeter et al. (2017) reported that the coherent breathing described in their study on the effect of Iyengar yoga on MDD optimizes HRV.

Neurotransmitters: Serotonin, Norepinephrine, and Dopamine

These three neurotransmitters – referred to collectively as monoamines – send signals between nerve cells and work in concert with one another. Serotonin is involved in the regulation of several processes within the brain, including mood, emotions, aggression, sleep, appetite, anxiety, memory, and perceptions (Telles et al., 2012). Norepinephrine acts as both a stress hormone – released from the adrenals into the blood during a stressful event – and a neurotransmitter. Dopamine has been thought to play a key role in pain processing, sleep, motor control, and metabolic regulation.

Yoga has been associated with increased norepinephrine neurotransmission, as well as serotonin synthesis and metabolism (Marefata et al., 2011). Meditative yoga practices have also been linked to serotonin and dopamine. When whole blood serotonin levels and mood state changes were assessed before and after *pranayama* in 15 participants, it was found that there was an increase in whole blood serotonin levels correlated with reduced negative feelings (Meyer et al., 2012). In a study of 67 meditators who had been practicing for 3–144 months and 57 non-meditators, the meditators had lower stress, higher positive affect, and higher plasma dopamine levels in comparison with the non-meditators (Telles et al., 2012).

GABA

The emotional balancing of yoga practices is related to an additional neurotransmitter: gamma aminobutyric acid (GABA). GABA is involved in the regulation of muscle excitability, sleep, and pain processing, and is associated with improved mood and decreased anxiety. Depression is related to lowered GABA levels in the cortex, and treatment with selective serotonin reuptake inhibitors (SSRIs), commonly prescribed anti-depression medications, has been found to be one way to increase GABA concentrations.

GABA levels have been shown to increase after yoga practice. In one study (Streeter et al., 2007), eight practitioners completed a 60-minute yoga session, and 11 non-practitioners read periodicals and popular fiction for 60 minutes. Using magnetic resonance spectroscopy imaging (MRSI), it was found that GABA levels had increased by 27% in the yoga group, while the control group showed no change. Furthermore, those who practiced more frequently and/or had been practicing for more years generally demonstrated the highest GABA levels. The second study by the same group (Streeter et al., 2010) took things a step further, exploring whether changes in GABA levels were specific to yoga or related to physical activity in general. Nineteen participants were randomized to a yoga group and 15 to a metabolically matched physical exercise group, and each practiced for 60 minutes, three times a week, for 12 weeks. Here again, MRSI demonstrated an increase in GABA levels in the yoga group over the control group; the yoga group also reported higher rates of mood improvement and anxiety symptom reduction.

BDNF

BDNF (brain-derived neurotrophic factor) is a protein thought to help support the survival of existing neurons and encourage the growth and differentiation of new ones. Studies suggest that both the aerobic (Meyer et al., 2012) and the meditative (Balasubramaniam, Telles, & Doraiswamy, 2012) components of yoga increase levels of BDNF.

Hormones: Cortisol and Melatonin

Cortisol and melatonin are two hormones secreted in the brain. You may be familiar with the role of cortisol, an important hormone that helps in dealing with stress. Equally crucial is melatonin, the anti-inflammatory, antioxidant hormone responsible for controlling sleep/wake cycles. Melatonin has been found to stimulate the immune system by acting as a powerful antioxidant, decrease blood pressure, stimulate the vagus nerve, and therefore reenergize the parasympathetic nervous system (Visceglia, 2015).

Just as it is associated with low HRV, depression is also associated with low levels of melatonin secretion (Meyer et al., 2012). Likewise, cortisol, produced in excess for those under chronic stress or whose bodies perceive them to be under chronic stress (i.e., as a result of chronic trauma), is associated at high levels with depression and connected with a hyperactive uptake of serotonin (Visceglia, 2015). Prolonged high cortisol levels are known to have many other adverse symptoms: lowered immunity, decreased bone density, decreased muscle tissue, and poor cognitive functioning (Douglass, 2011).

Studies have linked yoga to an increase in melatonin and a decrease in cortisol (Douglass, 2011; Meyer et al., 2012; Visceglia, 2015). Significantly higher levels of melatonin were observed in participants both immediately after they had completed yogic meditation sessions, as compared with control periods, and after a consistent three-month practice that included *asana, pranayama*, and meditation (*dhyana*). Brainard, Pratap, Reed, Levitt, and Hanifin (1997) found that participating in just one yoga class decreased cortisol levels. However, in one previously mentioned study of Iyengar yoga practices specifically for depression (Woolery et al., 2004), there was a trend in the yoga group controls for higher morning cortisol levels, which are associated with positive traits, as explained earlier.

Brain Structure and Activity

At times of emotional imbalance, several areas of the brain will function atypically. For example, during depression, abnormal functioning may be detected in 1) the anterior cingulate cortex, which includes regions involved in executive function, cognitive processes, and emotional regulation; and 2) prefrontal cortex areas involved in complex behaviors such as planning. In Chapter 2, we mentioned the National Institute of Mental Health longitudinal study of 389 children, in which reduction in volume of the brain's gray matter, frontal lobe, temporal lobe, and hippocampus were seen due to the effects of trauma.

The components of yoga have been shown to positively impact certain regions of the brain (Gard et al., 2014; Kinser et al., 2013; van der Kolk, 2006). For instance, one of the studies of chronically traumatized women with PTSD revealed that after 20 weeks of yoga, they had developed increased activation of the insula and the medial prefrontal cortex, critical brain structures involved in self-regulation (van der Kolk, 2015). This parallels some of the effects reported due to meditation practices on the brain, an area that has been studied in more depth: increased gray matter in the insula, hippocampus, and prefrontal cortex leading to improved attention, compassion, and empathy; reduced aging-related cortical thinning in prefrontal regions associated with attention, interoception, and sensory processing; and increased coherence and synchrony (ways in which different regions of the brain work together) leading to improved integrated brain functioning and problem-solving (Mendius & Hanson, 2009).

Evidence-Based Research versus Outcome-Based Therapy

Throughout this chapter, we have seen some promising research suggesting that yoga can indeed lead to a decrease in symptoms of emotional imbalance, whether these are assessed via self-report or biomarkers. However, it is important to note that results from such evidence-based research are very different from the work that you who are therapists would carry out with a client. What we have looked at in this chapter are studies that focus on streamlining and replicability: a measurement of the effects of a particular breath or posture series is far more effective in providing results that demonstrate the efficacy of yoga, and therefore facilitate its funding and inclusion in certain environments. When we are working with a client or on ourselves, on the other hand, we are more interested in a practice that is tailor-made and appropriate for that specific person's needs. That is the difference between evidence-based research and outcome-based therapy.

In outcome-based therapy (Laurence, 2010), "the use of research focuses on developing an individual or group practice that is based on local, individually obtained evidence through practice, rather than clinical studies" (p. 66). Other than for a few of the cases that we looked at earlier, namely Streeter et al.'s (2017) and Woolery's (2004) focus on Iyengar poses for depression, the LifeForce Yoga Program for depression (Bennett et al., 2008), the Trauma Center Trauma Sensitive Yoga programs for PTSD (e.g. Price et al., 2017; Rhodes et al., 2016; West et al., 2017; van der Kolk et al., 2014), and Shannahoff-Khalsa's (1999) inclusion of left nostril breathing for OCD symptoms, the protocols that we have seen in evidence-based research trials have not been specifically developed for the symptoms treated. Rather, participants are simply taking part in general population yoga practices.

Perhaps more importantly, evidence-based research typically lacks a significant element that we will be highlighting consistently in this book: relationship. That relationship may be between you as a therapist and your client, or it may be with yourself if you will be practicing with this book. Either way, it is a far more long-term, intimate relationship than the one in evidence-based research experiments. Especially when it comes to yoga, which may restore balance on the physical, emotional, mental, and spiritual levels, a richer, multifaceted relationship is key.

As Shorter points out, there are two "how" questions that we can ask about yoga. "The first question," she explains, "gets at how yoga works." That is the question we addressed in the previous pages. But it is actually the second question that Shorter highlights: "How do we use yoga to change people's lives?" (2013, p. 19). That question is the focus of the second half of this book. It describes and expands upon the Three-Pronged Model, providing practices that fit within the general framework but that nonetheless retain their individual orientation for each client. Let us now turn to that framework.

References

Alderman, B. L., Olson, R. L., Brush, C. J., & Shors, T. J. (2016). MAP training: Combining meditation and aerobic exercise reduces depression and rumination while enhancing synchronized brain activity. *Translational Psychiatry, 6*, e726. doi: 10.1038/tp.2015.225

Baer, R. A., Fischer, S., & Huss, D. B. (2005). Mindfulness-based cognitive therapy applied to binge eating: A case study. *Cognitive and Behavioral Practice, 12*(3), 351–8. doi: 10.1016/S1077-7229(05)80057-4

Balasubramaniam, M., Telles, S., & Doraiswamy, P. M. (2012). Yoga on our minds: A systematic review of yoga for neuropsychiatric disorders. *Frontiers in Psychiatry, 3*, 117. doi: 10.3389/fpsyt.2012.00117

Bennett, S. M., Weintraub, A., & Khalsa, S. B. (2008). Initial evaluation of the LifeForce Yoga Program as a therapeutic intervention for depression. *International Journal of Yoga Therapy, 18*, 49–57. Retrieved from https://yogafordepression.com/wp-content/uploads/initial-eval-of-lifeforce-yoga.pdf

Bock, B. C., Fava, J. L., Gaskins, R., Morrow, K. M., Williams, D. M., & Jennings, E. (2012). Yoga as a complementary treatment for smoking cessation in women. *Journal of Women's Health, 21*(2), 240–248. doi: 10.1089/jwh.2011.2963

Bowman, A. J., Clayton, R. H., Murray, A., Reed, J. W., Subhan, M. M., & Ford, G.A. (1997). Effects of aerobic exercise training and yoga on the baroreflex in healthy elderly persons. *European Journal of Clinical Investigation, 27*(5), 443–449. doi:10.1046/j.1365-2362.1997.1340681.x

Brainard, G., Pratap, V., Reed, C., Levitt, B., & Hanifin, J. (1997, April–September). Plasma control reduction in healthy volunteers following a single yoga session of yoga practices. *Yoga Research Society Newsletter*, No. 18.

Brisbon, N. M., & Lowery, G. A. (2011). Mindfulness and levels of stress: A comparison of beginner and advanced hatha yoga practitioners. *Journal of Religion and Health, 50*(4), 931–941. doi: 10.1007/s10943-009-9305-3

Burns, D., & Ohayv, R. J. (1980). Psychological changes in meditating Western monks in Thailand. *Journal of Transpersonal Psychology, 12*(1), 11–24. Retrieved from http://atpweb.org/jtparchive/trps-12-80-01-011.pdf

Butzer, B., Ahmed, K., & Khalsa, S. B. (2016). Yoga enhances positive psychological states in young adult musicians. *Applied Psychophysiology and Biofeedback, 41*(2), 191–202. doi: 10.1007/s10484-015-9321-x

Cabral, P., Meyer, H., & Ames, D. (2011). Effectiveness of yoga therapy as a complementary treatment for major psychiatric disorders: A meta-analysis. *The Primary Care Companion to CNS Disorders, 13*(4), PCC.10r01068. doi:10.4088/PCC.10r01068

Chen, K.-M., Chien, M.-H. C., Chao, H.-C., Hung, H.-M., Lin, H.-S., & Li, C.-H. L. (2009). Sleep quality, depression state, and health status of older adults after silver yoga exercises: Cluster randomized trial. *International Journal of Nursing Studies, 46*(2), 154–163. doi: 10.1016/j.ijnurstu.2008.09.005

Cramer, H., Lauche, R., Langhorst, J., & Dobos, G. (2013). Yoga for depression: A systematic review and meta-analysis. *Depression and Anxiety, 30*(11),1068–1083. doi: 10.1002/da.22166

da Silva, T. L., Ravindran, L. N., & Ravindran, A. V. (2009). Yoga in the treatment of mood and anxiety disorders: A review. *Asian Journal of Psychiatry, 2*(1), 6–16. doi: 10.1016/j.ajp.2008.12.002

Daubenmier, J. (2005). The relationship of yoga, body awareness, and body responsiveness to self-objectification and disordered eating. *Psychology of Women Quarterly, 29*(2), 207–219. doi: 10.1111/j.1471-6402.2005.00183.x

de Manincor, M., Bensoussan, A , Smith, C. A., Barr, K., Schweickle, M., Donoghoe, L.L., ... Fahey, P. (2016). Individualized yoga for reducing depression and anxiety, and improving well-being: A randomized controlled trial. *Depression and Anxiety, 33*(9), 816–828. doi: 10.1002/da.22502

Douglass, L. (2011). Thinking through the body: The conceptualization of yoga as therapy for individuals with eating disorders. *Eating Disorders, 19*(1), 83–96. doi: 10.1080/10640266.2011.533607

Duan-Porter, W., Coeytaux, R. R., McDuffie, J., Goode, A., Sharma, P., Mennella, H., ... Williams, J. W. (2016). Evidence map of yoga for depression, anxiety, and posttraumatic stress disorder. *Journal of Physical Activity & Health, 13*(3), 281–288. http://doi.org/10.1123/jpah.2015-0027

Elibero, A., Janse Van Rensburg, K., & Drobes, D. J. (2011). Acute effects of aerobic exercise and hatha yoga on craving to smoke. *Nicotine & Tobacco Research, 13*(11), 1140–1148. doi: 10.1093/ntr/ntr163

Field, T., Diego, M., and Hernandez-Reif, M. (2010). Tai chi/yoga effects on anxiety, heartrate, EEG and math computations. *Complementary Therapies in Clinical Practice, 16*(4), 235–238. doi: 10.1016/j.ctcp.2010.05.014

Follette, V., Palm, K., & Pearson, A. (2006). Mindfulness and trauma: Implications for treatment. *Journal of Rational-Emotive & Cognitive Behavior Therapy, 24*(1), 45–61. doi: 10.1007/s10942-006-0025-2

Fox, K. R. (1999). The influence of physical activity on mental well-being. *Public Health Nutrition, 2*(3a), 411–418. Retrieved from http://beauty-review.nl/wp-content/uploads/2015/03/The-influence-of-physical-activity-on-mental-well-being.pdf

Gard, T., Noggle, J. J., Park, C. D. R., & Wilson, A. (2014). Potential self-regulatory mechanisms of yoga for psychological health. *Frontiers in Human Neuroscience, 8*, 770. doi: 10.3389/fnhum.2014.00770

Gerbarg, P. L., & Brown, R. P. (2015). Yoga and neuronal pathways to enhance stress response: Emotion regulation, bonding, and spirituality. In E. G. Horovitz

& S. Elgelid (Eds.), *Yoga therapy: Theory and practice* (pp. 61–75). New York & London, Routledge.

Girodo, M. (1974). Yoga meditation and flooding in the treatment of anxiety neurosis. *Journal of Behavior Therapy and Experimental Psychiatry, 5*(2), 157–160. doi: 10.1016/0005-7916(74)90104-9

Grossman, P., Niemann, L., Schmidt, S., & Walach, H. (2004). Mindfulness-based stress reduction and health benefits. A meta-analysis. *Journal of Psychosomatic Research, 57*(1), 35–43. doi:10.1016/S0022-3999(03)00573-7

Hartfiel, N., Havenland, J., Khalsa, S. B., Clarke, G., & Krayer, A. (2011). The effectiveness of yoga for the improvement of well-being and resilience to stress in the workplace. *Scandinavian Journal of Work, Environment & Health, 37*(1), 70–76. www.jstor.org/stable/40967889

Jadhav, S. G., & Havalappanavar, N. B. (2009). Effect of yoga intervention on anxiety and subjective well-being. *Journal of the Indian Academy of Applied Psychology, 35*(1), 27–31. http://medind.nic.in/jak/t09/i1/jakt09i1p27.pdf

Javnbakht, M., Hejazi Kenari, R., & Ghasemi, M. (2009). Effects of yoga on depression and anxiety of women. *Complementary Therapies in Clinical Practice, 15*(2),102–104. doi: 10.1016/j.ctcp.2009.01.003

Johnston, J.M., Minami, T., Greenwald, D., Li, C., Reinhardt, K., & Khalsa S. B. (2015). Yoga for military service personnel with PTSD: A single arm study. *Psychological Trauma Theory Research, 7*(6), 555–562. doi: 10.1037/tra0000051

Kabat-Zinn, J. (2003). Mindfulness-based interventions in context: Past, present, and future. *Clinical Psychology: Science and Practice, 10*(2), 144–156. doi: 10.1093/clipsy.bpg016

Kalyani, B. G., Venkatasubramanian, G., Arasappa, R., Rao, N. P., Kalmady, S. V., Behere, R. V., ... Gangadhar, B. N. (2011). Neurohemodynamic correlates of "OM" chanting: A pilot functional magnetic resonance imaging study. *International Journal of Yoga, 4*(1), 3–6. doi: 10.4103/0973-6131.78171

Khalsa, S. B., & Cope, S. (2006). Effects of a yoga lifestyle intervention on performance-related characteristics of musicians: A preliminary study. *Medical Science Monitor, 12*(8), CR325-31.

Khalsa, S. B., Shorter, S. M., Cope, S., Wyshak, G., & Sklar, E. (2009). Yoga ameliorates performance anxiety and mood disturbance in young professional musicians. *Applied Psychophysiology Biofeedback, 34*(4), 279–289. doi: 10.1007/s10484-009-9103-4

Kimbrough, E., Magyari, T., Langenberg, P., Chesney, M., & Berman, B. (2010). Mindfulness intervention for child abuse survivors. *The Journal of Clinical Psychology, 66*(1), 17–33. doi: 10.1002/jclp.20624

Kinser, P. A., Bourgignon, C., Whaley, D., Hauenstein, E., & Taylor, A. G. (2013). Feasibility, acceptability, and effects of gentle hatha yoga for women with major depression: Findings from a randomized controlled mixed-methods study. *Archives of Psychiatric Nursing, 27*(3), 137–147. doi: 10.1016/j.apnu.2013.01.003

Kirkwood, G., Rampes, H., Tuffrey, V., Richardson, J., & Pilkington, K. (2005). Yoga for anxiety: A systematic review of the research evidence. *British Journal of Sports Medicine, 39*(12), 884–891. doi:10.1136/bjsm.2005.018069

Kreher, S. (2015). Yoga for anger management. In E. G. Horovitz & S. Elgelid (Eds.), *Yoga therapy: Theory and Practice* (pp. 172–184). New York & London: Routledge.

Laurence, S. (2010). Issues in yoga therapy: The role of outcome-based standards in yoga therapy. *International Journal of Yoga Therapy, 20*(1), 65–71. Retrieved June 21, 2018, from: https://yogafordepression.com/wp-content/uploads/the-role-of-outcome-based-standards-in-yoga-therapy-scott-laurence.pdf

Lavey, R., Sherman, T., Mueser, K. T., Osborne, D. D., Currier, M., & Wolfe, R. (2005). The effects of yoga on mood in psychiatric inpatients. *Psychiatric Rehabilitation Journal, 28*(4), 399–402. doi:10.2975/28.2005.399.402

Levine, M. (2009). *The positive psychology of Buddhism and yoga: Paths to a mature happiness*. New York & London: Routledge.

Lilly, M., & Hedlund, J. (2010). Yoga therapy in practice: Healing childhood sexual abuse with yoga. *International Journal of Yoga Therapy, 20*, 120–130. Retrieved from https://yogafordepression.com/wp-content/uploads/healing-childhood-sexual-abuse-with-yoga-lilly-and-hedlund.pdf

Lin, P., Chang, J., Zemon, V., & Milarsky, E. (2008). Silent illumination: A study on Chan (Zen) meditation, anxiety, and musical performance quality. *Psychology of Music, 36*(2), 139–155. doi:10.1177/0305735607080840

Marefata, M., Peymanzad, H., & Alikhajeh, Y. (2011). Study of the effects of yoga exercises on addicts' depression and anxiety in rehabilitation. *Social and Behavioral Sciences, 30*, 1494–1498. https://doi.org/10.1016/j.sbspro.2011.10.289

McIver, S., O'Halloran, P., & McGartland, M. (2009). Yoga as a treatment for binge eating disorder: A preliminary study. *Complementary Therapies in Medicine, 17*(4), 196–202. doi: 10.1016/j.ctim.2009.05.002

Mehta, P., & Sharma, M. (2010). Yoga as a complementary therapy for clinical depression. *Complementary Health Practice Review, 15*(3), 156–170. doi: 10.1177/1533210110387405

Mendius, R., & Hanson, R. (2009). *Buddha's brain: The practical neuroscience of happiness, love & wisdom*. Oakland, CA: New Harbinger Publications.

Meyer, H. B., Katsman, A., Sones, A. C., Auerbach, D. E., Ames, D., & Rubin, R. T. (2012). Yoga as an ancillary treatment for neurological and psychiatric disorders: A review. *Journal of Neuropsychiatry and Clinical Neurosciences, 24*(2), 152–164. doi: 10.1176/appi.neuropsych.11040090

Mitchell, K. S., Dick, A. M., DiMartino, D. M., Smith, B. N., Niles, B., Koenen, K. C., & Street, A. (2014). A pilot study of a randomized controlled trial of yoga as an intervention for PTSD symptoms in women. *Journal of Traumatic Stress, 27*(2), 121–128. doi: 10.1002/jts.21903

Mitchell, K. S., Mazzeo, S. E., Rausch, S. M., & Cooke, K. L. (2007). Innovative interventions for disordered eating: Evaluating dissonance-based and yoga interventions. *International Journal of Eating Disorders, 40*(2), 120–128. doi:10.1002/eat.20282

Netz, Y., & Lidor, R. (2003). Mood alterations in mindful versus aerobic exercise modes. *Journal of Psychology, 137*(5), 405–419. doi:10.1080/00223980309600624

Pilkington, K., Kirkwood, G., Rampes, H., & Richardson, J. (2005). Yoga for depression: The research evidence. *Journal of Affective Disorders, 89*, 13–24. doi: 10.1016/j.jad.2005.08.013

Price, M., Spinazzola, J., Musicaro, R., Turner, J., Suvak, M., Emerson, D., & van der Kolk, B. A. (2017). Effectiveness of an extended yoga treatment for women with chronic posttraumatic stress disorder. *Journal of Alternative and Complementary Medicine, 23*(4), 300–309. doi: 10.1089/acm.2015.0266

Reibel, D., Greeson, J., Brainard, G., & Rosenzwig, S. (2001). Mindfulness-based stress reduction and health-related quality of life in a heterogeneous patient population. *General Hospital Psychiatry, 23*(4),183–192. doi:10.1016/S0163-8343(01)00149-9

Rhodes, A. (2015). Claiming peaceful embodiment through yoga in the aftermath of trauma. *Complementary Therapies in Clinical Practice, 21*(4), 247–256. doi: 10.1016/j.ctcp.2015.09.004

Rhodes, A., Spinazzola, J., & van der Kolk, B. (2016). Yoga for adult women with chronic PTSD: A long-term follow-up study. *The Journal of Alternative and Complementary Medicine, 22*(3), 189–196. doi:10.1089/acm.2014.0407

Ross, A., and Thomas, S. (2010). The health benefits of yoga and exercise: A review of comparison studies. *Journal of Alternative & Complementary Medicine, 16*(1), 3–12. doi: 10.1089/acm.2009.0044

Ross, A., Bevans, M., Friedmann, E., Williams, L., & Thomas, S. (2014). "I am a nice person when I do yoga!!!" A qualitative analysis of how yoga affects relationships. *Journal of Holistic Nursing American Holistic Nurses Association, 32*(2), 67–77. doi: 10.1177/0898010113508466

Shannahoff-Khalsa, D. S., Ray, L. E., Levine, S., Gallen, C. C., Schwartz, B. J., & Sidorowish, J. (1999). Randomized controlled trial of yogic meditation techniques for patients with obsessive-compulsive disorder. *CNS Spectrums, 4*(12), 34–47. doi: 10.1017/S1092852900006805

Shorter, S. M. (2013) Yoga at the intersection of research and service – part 1: Experimental foundations. *Journal of Yoga Service, 1*(1): 15–22. Retrieved from https://yogafordepression.com/wp-content/uploads/Yoga-at-the-Intersection-of-Research.pdf

Streeter, C. C., Gerbarg, P. L., Saper, R. B., Ciraulo, D. A., & Brown R. P. (2012) Effects of yoga on the autonomic nervous system, gamma-aminobutyric-acid, and allostasis in epilepsy, depression, and post-traumatic stress disorder. *Medical Hypotheses, 78*(5), 571–579. doi: 10.1016/j.mehy.2012.01.021.

Streeter, C. C., Gerbarg, P. L., Whitfield, T. H., Owen, L., Johnston, J., Silveri, M. M., … Jensen, J. E. (2017). Treatment of major depressive disorder with Iyengar yoga and coherent breathing: A randomized controlled dosing study. *Journal of Alternative and Complementary Medicine, 23*(3), 201–207. doi: 10.1089/acm.2016.0140

Streeter, C. C., Jensen, J. E., Perlmutter, R. M., Cabral, H. J., Tian, H., Terhune, D. B., … Renshaw, P. F. (2007) Yoga asana sessions increase brain GABA levels: A pilot study. *The Journal of Alternative and Complementary Medicine, 13*(4), 419–426. doi:// 10.1089/acm.2007.6338

Streeter, C. C., Whitfield, T. H., Owen, L., Rein, T., Karri, S., Yakhkind, A., … Jensen, J. E. (2010). Effects of yoga versus walking on mood, anxiety, and brain GABA levels: A randomized controlled MRS study. *Journal of Alternative & Complementary Medicine, 16*(11), 1145–1152. doi: 10.1089/acm.2010.0007

Ströhle, A. (2009). Physical activity, exercise, depression and anxiety disorders. *Journal of Neural Transmission, 116*(6), 777–784. doi: 10.1007/s00702-008-0092-x

Sullivan, M. B., Erb, M., Schmalzl, L., Moonaz, S., Taylor, J. N., & Porges, S. W (2018). Yoga therapy and polyvagal theory: The convergence of traditional wisdom and contemporary neuroscience for self-regulation and resilience. *Frontiers in Human Neuroscience, 12*, 67. doi: 10.3389/fnhum.2018.00067

Telles, S., Singh, N., & Balkrishna, A. (2012). Managing mental health disorders resulting from trauma through yoga: A review. *Depression Research and Treatment, 2012,* 401513. doi:10.1155/2012/401513

Uebelacker, L. A., & Broughton, M. K. (2016). Yoga for depression and anxiety: A review of published research and implications for healthcare providers. *Rhode Island Medical Journal, 99*(3), 20–22. doi:10.1176/appi.focus.16104

Uebelacker, L. A., Weinstock, L., & Kraines, M. (2014). Self-reported benefits and risks of yoga in individuals with bipolar disorder. *Journal of Psychiatric Practice, 20*(5), 345–352. doi: 10.1097/01.pra.0000454779.59859.f8

van der Kolk, B. A. (2006). Clinical implications of neuroscience research in PTSD. *Annals of the New York Academy of Sciences, 1071,* 277–293. http://dx.doi.org/10.1196/annals.1364.022

van der Kolk, B. A. (2015). *The body keeps the score: Brain, mind, and body in the healing of trauma.* New York, NY: Penguin Books.

van der Kolk, B. A., Stone, L., West, J., Rhodes, A., Emerson, D., Suvak, M., & Spinazzola, J. (2014). Yoga as an adjunctive treatment for posttraumatic stress disorder: A randomized controlled trial. *The Journal of Clinical Psychiatry, 75*(6), e559–65. doi: 10.4088/JCP.13m08561

Varambally, S., Vidyendaran, S., Sajjanar, M., Thirthalli, J., Hamza, A., Nagendra, H. R., & Gangadhar, B. N. (2013). Yoga-based intervention for caregivers of outpatients with psychosis: A randomized controlled pilot study. *Asian Journal of Psychiatry, 6*(2), 141–145. doi: 10.1016/j.ajp.2012.09.017

Visceglia, E. (2015). Psychiatry and yoga therapy. In L. Payne, T. Gold, E. Goldman, & C. Rosenberg (Eds.), *Yoga therapy & integrative medicine: Where ancient science meets modern medicine* (pp. 143–155). Laguna Beach, CA: Basic Health Publications, Inc.

West, J., Liang, B., & Spinazzola, J. (2017). Trauma sensitive yoga as a complementary treatment for posttraumatic stress disorder: A qualitative descriptive analysis. *International Journal of Stress Management, 24*(2), 173–195. doi:10.1037/str0000040

Woolery, A., Myers, H., Sternlieb, B., & Zeltzer, L. (2004). A yoga intervention for young adults with elevated symptoms of depression. *Alternative Therapies in Health and Medicine, 10*(2), 60–63. Retrieved from www.aeyt.org/resources/A%20yoga%20intervention%20for%20young%20adults%20with%20elevated%20symptoms%20of%20depression.pdf

Part II
Application

4 Beginning the Practice

Welcome to Part II, the applied portion of this book. Now that we have more of an understanding of yoga, emotional health, and some of the research on the intersection of the two, we can move forward with working with the Three-Pronged Model. The first part of this chapter raises important points to consider before embarking on a yoga journey with a client, while the second focuses on starting that journey. Some of these elements are helpful to consider for any beginning therapist, whereas others are specific to working with yoga, and so are beneficial to consider even for therapists experienced in other modalities.

While this chapter is mainly intended for the therapist, it will still be of benefit to you if you are reading this book with an eye to turning to yoga for your own emotional balance. It may give you insight into assessing your own readiness and progression, as well as what to look for in a therapist should you decide to work with one in the future.

Before Meeting Your Client

Your Intention

In Chapter 1, we talked about *sankalpa*, or intention, in the context of a yoga practice. Intention is also one of the most important aspects to assess before you start working in any healing profession. People are drawn to the helping professions for many different reasons. They may feel a calling to assist in relieving others' suffering and helping them heal from their emotional wounds. Or they may feel that caring for others brings a sense of purpose and meaning to their own lives. Why did *you* choose a journey within this profession? If you are a yoga therapist, what interests you in working with emotional health in particular? If you are a psychotherapist, what is leading you to yoga as a modality? Sit with these questions, and notice your responses to them. Just observe.

Your Role

Sometimes, people turn to therapy because they want to tell others what
to do. I remember when I was in graduate school, several of my classmates
said something along the lines of, "People told me I should become a
therapist because I give good advice." My first psychotherapy mentor,
whom I have previously mentioned in Chapter 2, rapidly disabused me of
the notion that this facilitates healing or empowerment. He consistently
highlighted the importance of the "I–thou" relationship, the one in which
therapist and client co-create a personal encounter as two human beings.
In that encounter, the therapist is simply a guide on a journey, privileging
the client's inner wisdom over his own ego. That is what nurtures healing
and empowerment.

Stefan Elgelid (2015) distinguishes between two models of care. The
first is the medical model, which, he explains,

> is based on the idea that medical care is given for an illness or injury.
> The medical practitioner administers the treatment to the patient. The
> illness or injury will be cured/healed and the patient will be declared
> well ... The educational component often consists of the therapist
> instructing the patient in certain exercises. The patient demonstrates
> an understanding of the exercises and will continue to perform the
> exercises until full, or optimal health is reached. The patient will leave
> the medical model with better health status on the measures that
> relate to the illness or injury, but the patient does not have a deeper
> knowledge of his or her self and usually acts, feels, and thinks the same
> way as he did before the illness.
>
> (pp. 119–120)

The second is the educational model, which, on the other hand,

> comes from the word Educere – to bring out or draw out. A good
> education "draws out" what is already there. From a yoga perspective
> it is about helping the client draw out information/knowledge that is
> already present in the client. The goal is to get the client to mobilize
> his or her own resources. The yoga therapist can guide and facilitate the
> process, but the client is using the resources that are already present in
> him or her. The educational model is an *interactive* approach and both the
> practitioner and client stand to benefit and learn from the interaction.
>
> (p. 120, emphasis mine)

"The bottom line," expands Elgelid,

> is that we need to meet our clients where they are, where we are,
> and provide them with the guidance that they need for a successful

outcome. If the medical model is an appropriate starting point, then that is where we start but we can gently guide our clients towards the educational model so that in the future they will have more self-awareness and will be less likely to have the same problem again. If the educational model is the starting point, then that is where we start and we guide the client towards where they need to go from there.

(p. 128)

Our role is not to "fix" the client's symptoms from an all-knowing position from above, but to provide guidance towards inner knowledge from our place as a co-traveler in their journey. For instance, I may guide someone to turn right and he may decide to turn left instead. If I am insistent that he should have turned right, I am not honoring his inner knowledge. Now, if he requests guidance again, I am not in a place to guide him, as I am ignorant of his needs. If, however, I am curious about why he wanted to turn left instead, now I am learning about him, and can guide him more effectively if he requests further guidance in the future.

Sometimes therapists' lack of attunement is due to an assumption that their client will feel the same effects from certain practices as they themselves have in the past. If I make a statement to a client such as, "Now we're going to do a pose that will be calming," or "Now we'll come into a nice stretch," I am imposing my own experience – or that of others I have witnessed – on that student. These are statements that highlight attachment to outcome. By determining outcome, we are denying the central importance of the client's inner awareness, which is the crux of healing and wholeness. As David Emerson (2015) questions, what, then, happens to the role of interoception?

Making assumptions regarding a client's experience reduces treatment to a simple relationship between a disorder and a prescribed yogic treatment, working with what Scott Laurence in his discussion of outcome-based therapy describes as a "means," rather than an "ends," approach. A "means" approach, explains Laurence (2010, p. 69), "might insist that a therapist know a specific number of *asanas*, or Sanskrit terms, or anatomical concepts," whereas in an "ends" approach, expertise is "measured by how real clients assess the therapy's effectiveness, regardless of what the therapist knows or has achieved." Researcher and yoga teacher Laura Douglass (2011, p. 92) expresses this poignantly, highlighting that while we have made gains in discovering more about the science of yoga's effectiveness, neuroscience "still may not hold all the answers. Each human experience of suffering is a *unique and disordered confluence* of biological distress, personality, and cultural demands colliding to create feelings of isolation, fear, and terror" (italics mine). Such strong emotions are what lead some of our clients to seek our help, and it is irresponsible then for us simply to reduce such complexity to a diagnosis and its "solution."

In previous chapters, we talked about "beginner's mind" – approaching each practice as if it were your first. How will you cultivate beginner's mind as a therapist, so that you approach each client with a sense of curiosity? How will you allow yourself to be truly present and witness the journey, instead of attempting to control it? How will you relate to the dynamic between you and the client not as a hierarchy, but as a *relationship*?

Your Comfort Level

It is crucial to tune into your comfort level as you prepare to engage with clients. If you are a yoga therapist, are you at ease with the subject of emotional health? If you are a psychotherapist, are you comfortable with the elements of yoga that you are introducing? It is understandable to be a little nervous when trying out something new, but if your nervousness is palpable to your client, that does not create a safe space.

Second, to which populations are you drawn to work, and with whom are you nervous to work? It is important to operate within your scope of competence, which refers to the areas of practice a particular therapist is able, experienced, or expert in providing. Scope of competence is individual, based on the therapist's education, training, and experience, in contrast with scope of practice – discussed later – which refers to what is appropriate in the profession as a whole.

When we are uncomfortable, we tend not to be present. We live in mind chatter, which may lead us to vacillate between fear and recklessness. Notice if you spend much of your time before a session being agitated (*ksipta*) or checked out/blasé (*viksipta*) in order not to feel the fear. If you are noticing these responses, pay closer attention to whether your fear is rising from inexperience, or from a mismatch between the skills needed and your skills. Would training in those skills help you, or would that particular aspect of work feel ill-fitting to you?

Your Deliverable

You may have been told in a past marketing context to come up with a one-minute elevator speech describing what you do. While you may not go for that option (I like to emphasize different aspects of what I do depending on my audience, for example), it is important to be clear in your mind about what you offer.

One of the challenges of emotional health work is that it can be hard to quantify in terms of positive gain. We can talk about feeling "less anxious" or "less depressed," but what exactly does that mean? In my view, what we are offering when focusing on emotional health is an experience, not an outcome. I tend to explain to clients that we will be working with some yoga practices and exploring how they will affect the emotions.

I also highlight that we all experience things differently, and therefore every journey that a client and I embark on is its own voyage of discovery. The International Association of Yoga Therapists points out in its scope of practice (2016),

> The yoga tradition views each human being as a multidimensional system that includes numerous aspects – including body, breath, and mind (intellect and emotions) – and their mutual interaction. Yoga therapy is founded on the basic principle that intelligent practice can positively influence the direction of change within these human dimensions, *which are distinct from an individual's unchanging nature or spirit.*
>
> (p. 2, emphasis mine)

As psychiatrist Elizabeth Visceglia (2015) points out,

> Strikingly, even the same group Yoga practice seems to affect individuals differently ... therapeutic Yoga practice has both the generalized positive effects ... as well as particular individual effects that are often subtler and more difficult to predict at the outset of treatment.
>
> (pp. 147–148)

So I emphasize experience, and I *never* promise outcomes. A client who calls yearning for healing would love to hear that I can deliver, and my ego is strongly drawn to a reassurance that I will. But liability issues aside, I am not a fortune teller. I can describe what has already happened, not try to predict what will happen. So I can share that others have found relief in their therapeutic yoga practices, and at the same time, I can explain that just as the path to where this potential client is now was an individual one, so the journey from here will be too.

Yoga Therapist: Your Scope of Practice and Role as a Complementary Practitioner

As opposed to scope of competence, which signifies a therapist's individual education, training, and experience, scope of practice refers to a set of guidelines and parameters for the profession. A yoga therapist focusing on emotional health needs to be cognizant of how her education, training, and experience differ from those of a psychotherapist. As the IAYT Standards (2016) point out, a

> yoga therapist is NOT qualified to:
>   Undertake individual or group psychological counselling, unless appropriately qualified to do so ...

Diagnose a medical or psychological condition, unless qualified to do so as a licensed healthcare practitioner.

Advise clients about ceasing medication prescribed by another healthcare practitioner, unless qualified to do so as a licensed healthcare practitioner.

Make recommendations regarding the advice or treatment provided by another healthcare professional, unless appropriately qualified to do so.

(pp. 3, 4, 5)

One of the most important elements I always highlight to yoga therapists is that your role is a complementary one. As passionate as you might be about the impact of yoga, it is outside of your scope of practice to suggest it as the sole source of healing for a client. For example, we see from the preceding guidelines that it is highly unethical to suggest that someone stop their medication because they have started therapeutic yoga. If a client asks you about that, you should unequivocally refer them to a physician for assessment.

Your Boundaries

Scope of practice is part of the general category of boundaries about which it is crucial to gain clarity before starting to see clients. Notice your patterns regarding boundaries in your life in general. Many of us can be too rigid or too loose with them. We can be closed off and unwelcoming, or too eager to please. Some of us maintain similar boundary patterns throughout the different aspects of our lives, whereas others can have clear boundaries at work and murky ones in our personal lives, for example.

Maintaining boundaries can be a challenging area, especially in the helping professions. There can be an expectation that you should help anyone at any time. But providing clear boundaries around role and availability is healthy and helpful for clients, as it clarifies expectations. Do you respond to calls and emails between sessions? Is there a maximum beyond which you will not respond? What are your business hours, and are you available outside of them? What is your cancellation policy? What should a client do in an emergency? Most psychotherapists' voicemails direct a client in an emergency to hang up and dial 911 and/or the number for a local crisis hotline.

On your end as the therapist, you need to have a clear sense of what you need in order to preserve your energy. If your boundaries become murky and you begin responding to client requests during hours or with a frequency that is inappropriate for you, you will find yourself in the long run becoming depleted and building resentment.

Boundary issues also come up when you want to be closer to students. Unfortunately, the yoga world has been rocked by manifold instances of unhealthy teacher–student boundaries. While many of these have been sexual, unclear boundaries are not necessarily sexual. They can come up any time the relationship between teacher/therapist and student/client slides into something else. Likewise, inappropriate therapist–client relationships are hardly unheard of in the psychotherapy world, even though dual or multiple relationships are prohibited for psychotherapists.

Dual or multiple relationship is a situation in which multiple roles exist between a therapist and a client. For example, I have had several clients invite me to holiday parties, and I always decline. Why is it a good idea to decline? Let's say I go, and I break my client's favorite vase. Let's say I go, and my client's sister takes a dislike to me for some reason, and shares this dislike with my client. Could either of those events affect the relationship between my client and me? Absolutely. My relationship with my client is far more important than my attending one more holiday party. Avoiding dual relationship is wise regardless of whether you are a psychotherapist or a yoga therapist.

Even when therapists and clients keep their relationship within the therapy room, their involvement in intensive therapeutic work can lead to unhealthy psychological dependencies. Sometimes, clients project onto their therapists expectations that transgress the appropriate role, and therapists – if they have their own unexamined unmet needs – may find themselves feeding into these unhealthy bonds. A therapist who wished to become a parent and was unable to may find herself becoming overly attached to and emotionally dependent on her younger clients, for instance. Worse still, therapists might seek to exploit their students' vulnerability for personal ego gratification. That is one more reason why focusing on client self-empowerment is key.

Your Readiness

Now that you've assessed these elements, it is time to revisit a central question: are you ready to embark on this journey? You do not want to start with a client and then find that you had not in fact been ready, and bow out. If that ends up having to happen, it is not the end of the world as long as you handle it appropriately, but you want to be as sure as you can be that there are no clear obstacles on this path for you. Really sit in stillness with yourself, and notice what is happening internally. Notice sensations in your body as you envision yourself working with yoga and emotional health. Notice your breath. Then, notice what thoughts come up.

Starting with the Client

Meeting the Client

You decide you are ready to embark on your work with therapeutic yoga, and now it is time to see your first client. The first important thing to keep in mind is where you meet them energetically. If I am working with a client with depression who enters in a state of *mudha*, listless and with a flat affect, and I – whether inadvertently or because I want to lift his mood – start chatting brightly, my client will not be ready to join me there. The energy will feel jarring to him. Rather, I need to notice where he is, and then start just a tiny step above his energy level. If his voice is very slow and low, mine is just a fraction less slow, a hair less low. If he is not ready to answer questions and is more comfortable sitting in silence, I may invite him to sit in silence, adding a slight engagement with the breath, minor attention to the straightness of the spine. I will start from where he is, and make just a tiny adjustment.

Establishing Safety

Jim Hopper, an expert on sexual abuse and mindfulness at Harvard Medical School, has described "establishing safety and stability in one's body, one's relationships, and the rest of one's life" as an essential step in healing (Lilly & Hedlund, 2010, p. 121). Creating safety in the therapeutic context is the first step to that.

Safety in the therapeutic space comes in many forms. The central one is via a therapeutic alliance that encourages openness and acceptance, so that the client does not feel ashamed, fearful, or defensive when sharing information, including feedback about practices she is finding ineffective. While we may not be able to control judgmental thoughts since we are human, we can control our words and actions. We want to ensure that our clients feel free to be vulnerable without fear of repercussion.

There are several other important aspects to safety. One is preserving clear boundaries, as discussed earlier. Another is maintaining confidentiality, especially in small yoga communities where news can spread like wildfire: you will never share what the client says, unless it has to do with potential harm to self and/or others, or unless you need to engage in consultation with a more experienced therapist. Finally, check in with yourself consistently to make sure that you are doing your due diligence as a therapist, carrying out an informed assessment and devising a thoughtful, appropriate plan of care for your client.

Explaining What You Do

The first session is the chance to outline our approach to the client. The more clearly we lay things out at the onset, the more informed and therefore empowered she is, and the more able we are to progress smoothly. There are four themes that I especially like to emphasize from the start:

- The client is the ultimate judge of what is appropriate for his body. What I am offering are suggestions.

- Throughout our practice, we will continuously be bringing the attention back to the body and physical sensations. Whenever we are tempted to go to the story, we will return to the body. In the words of David Emerson (2015), founder of Trauma Sensitive Yoga, "there is no attempt to make meaning out of a body experience" (p. 13). The minute we endeavor to do that, we have moved away from the physical and into the cognitive, creating distance from the felt experience and privileging certain interpretations over others. The story about what happened is not the present; the physical sensations in the moment are the present.

- We will be approaching the body with a spirit of curiosity. As yoga teacher Natasha Rizopoulos (2017) highlights, not only are you in a flow of poses or practices, but "you're also in a flow with yourself" (p. 84). Each day, hour, and minute you experience is different in some shape or form. You may recall that in our discussion of the psychosocial benefits of yoga in Chapter 3, the flow of experience in the practice was ultimately one of the most helpful elements in emotional healing.

- As the client and I work together, I will do regular check-ins where I will ask for one word that describes how her body is feeling in the moment. Again, that word is about the present-moment physical sensation, not its interpretation or story, however tempting those directions might be. The word is the first one that comes to mind. I highlight that although sometimes people are tempted to start thinking of a word before I ask, that will actually detract from the benefit of the practice. It is fine if the client repeats the same word at different times if that is what he is feeling. Finally, I emphasize how important it is for the client to honestly report whatever physical sensations and emotions arise, rather than what she thinks I want to hear.

Gathering Information

One of the skills that you will develop as you work with yoga is how to cull the appropriate relevant information, without gathering too little or too much. The drawbacks of collecting too little information are apparent, but too much also can pose challenges. One is that it may imply a scope of practice that is inaccurate; for example, that may occur if you ask questions about nutrition habits and you do not have additional expertise in that area. Another is that you can overgeneralize details that may reflect only a moment in time; for instance, your client may report a mood at intake that you take to be reflective of how he always feels.

At the end of this chapter is an intake form with ten questions that I find useful when embarking on a journey of yoga for emotional health. Please note that this form focuses only on specific emotional health elements, and is not meant to be a comprehensive intake form. These are sample questions that you might consider adding to whatever intake you already carry out as a psychotherapist or yoga therapist. For a thorough sample of intake forms for yoga therapy, see Ellen Horovitz's examples in the appendices to *Yoga Therapy: Theory and Practice* (2015).

I would like to comment briefly on four pieces of intake information that I think are imperative for you to collect:

- Medical information, including medical providers' names, all diagnoses and who gave them, surgeries, medication, and clearance to begin a yoga therapy program if the client has a serious condition. Ask specifically how each of the conditions affects the client day-to-day. You are doing your best to assess for any risk factors or contraindications.

Do not let a client leave the medical provider category blank. If something happens, you need to be able to have someone to contact. If the client insists he does not have a physician, have the name of a physician or facility handy, and let the client know this will be who you will contact in case of a medical or psychiatric emergency (including potential self-harm if you are a yoga therapist). If the client has a medical provider, ask for permission to speak with that person; for an example of a release form to do that, see Horovitz (2015), Appendix B.

- Sources of support, whether these are friends, spiritual figures, or otherwise. Ask directly if you can use them as emergency contacts, in addition to any others whom the client may have listed at intake. Make sure that the client has received permission from these people to be contacted in an emergency – you do not want to make a call at that time to a person who is not ready to help. If you are a yoga therapist, also let your client know that you will contact these people if you feel there is a risk for any sort of self-harm. If you are a psychotherapist, you would follow the procedure you typically follow regarding self-harm potential.
- Information from any client who has previously practiced yoga on what she has found helpful in her practice, as well as her favorite pose and the reason behind that choice. Beyond giving you a basis on which to build, it also tells you more about the emotional state at which the client is hoping to arrive. If the client on her intake form gives you a reason that sounds physical (for example, "I like wheel pose because it makes me feel strong"), remember that the physical holds the key to the emotional.
- Three measurable goals that will indicate to the client down the road that she is beginning to shift emotionally. These goals should be clear and concise, and you will derive them from the primary reasons for coming to yoga therapy that the client has written on the intake form. For example, if she wrote, "I want to feel less depressed," you would proceed as follows towards a measurable goal:

THERAPIST: What would be one thing you would be doing if you were less depressed?

CLIENT: Seeing my friends more.

THERAPIST: How frequently do you see them now?

CLIENT: I don't.

THERAPIST: So if you started feeling a little less depressed, how frequently would you see them?

CLIENT: I used to see them twice a week.

THERAPIST: Ok. You used to see them twice a week, and now you don't see them. If you started feeling a little less depressed, how frequently do you think you would see them?

CLIENT: Maybe once a week.

THERAPIST: Shall we say then that one of the ways you would be able to see that things have begun to shift emotionally is that you would see your friends once a week?

CLIENT: Ok.

Notice that the therapist here kept his eyes on the prize: a clear, concise statement that could serve as an indication of change.

Assessing Readiness

Just as we observed our own readiness to embark on the journey of yoga therapy, so we need to assess our clients'. Just because someone is ready for talk therapy, that does not necessarily mean that they are prepared for yoga. Somatically oriented therapies are powerful in their effectiveness, but in order for progress to occur, the client has to be willing potentially to experience strong bodily emotions. As Bessel van der Kolk points out (2015), "As long as we register emotions primarily in our heads we can remain pretty much in control, but feeling as if our chest is caving in or we've been punched in the gut is unbearable" (p. 276). We want to make sure our clients are aware that accessing emotions via the body can be very different from talking about them. At the same time, it is our responsibility to guide their experience in a way that keeps them with dual attention and within their window of tolerance, two concepts discussed later.

Part of assessing readiness for a practice is assessing *what* someone is ready for. I may be ready to approach working with my depression gingerly, but not to delve deeply into it. We assume that emotional release is cathartic, but while that can be the case, it is not always so. Sometimes we become scared of our intense emotions, and it would have been wiser to use a more cautious approach. There is nothing that will shatter a sense of safety more than when a client feels that her emotions are spiraling out of control, and the therapist's assertion that "that's part of the process" may not necessarily be reassuring (or true).

I cannot emphasize enough that when it comes to emotional health, readiness is about stability. Assessing readiness means evaluating stability. In yoga we are very fond of "going inside," but when "inside" is filled with dark, tumultuous emotions, the client may not want to be there. For other clients, their traumas are so severe that they are not in the here and now, but live inside the heightened emotions of the trauma, and need practice emerging from there. The key to healing is dual attention: being aware of the world around you as well as the feelings within you.

Another way of saying this is that you need to assess your client's capacity for exteroception and interoception. Exteroception refers to outward orientation, and receiving direct information from the external environment. It is what detects and informs us of the external environment via the senses of sight, hearing, smell, taste, and touch. Interoception, as we defined briefly in Chapter 3, refers to the awareness of the internal state of one's body. It detects and informs us of such internal regulation responses as respiration, heart rate, body temperature, balance, hunger/ thirst, need for digestive elimination, emotions, and pleasure/pain. Those who struggle with interoceptive sense may have trouble knowing when they feel hungry, full, hot, cold, or thirsty. Having trouble with this sense can also make self-regulation a challenge.

Exteroception

Assessing readiness begins with exteroception. It is easier to shift back to the external if your client is flooded by the internal experience than to try to introduce it for the first time while the flooding is occurring. To orient externally, I have come to use the "54321" approach, a common grounding technique in psychotherapy. I explain to the client that part of the journey of shifting from the overwhelm of emotions is to guide ourselves into the here and now, and that this technique helps us to do that. I invite the client to sit comfortably, then I guide her using the italicized words below.

Look around the room. Say out loud:

- *5 things that you see*
- *4 things that you're touching, or are touching you*
- *3 things that you hear*
- *2 things that you smell*
- *1 taste in your mouth*

From Exteroception to Interoception

From here, I will now invite a shift from the outside to the inside, which I base on a technique used in Somatic Experiencing.

Now look around the room, and allow your eyes to land on something that pleases you.

Notice what it is in your body that indicates to you that it pleases you.

In addition to alerting you to your client's awareness of internal sensations, this practice demonstrates to you the ease with which the client can access emotions that are less intense. We may feel tightness in the chest or butterflies in the stomach, but are we able to detect opening in the chest or easing in the stomach? A client who answers your prompt of "Notice what it is in your body that indicates to you that it pleases you" with "I don't know" may not be as tuned in to subtle internal shifts, and therefore is a person with whom you want to proceed slowly. She may respond to check-ins with "I feel fine," and not be aware of emotional shifts until they are large and potentially overwhelming.

Grounding Posture

Now that we have assessed the client's senses of exteroception and interoception, we will introduce movement and see how that is for the client. The Mountain pose through which I will guide the client here involves quite a few directions, as my purpose is to orient him to the body, and to the here and now.

MOUNTAIN POSE

Come to standing, with your feet hip-width apart. In order to identify hip-width, find the front of your hip bones and line each up with the second toe of that foot. Bring your arms by your sides.

Spread the toes wide. Shift your weight forward to the front of your feet, towards the toes. Shift your weight backwards to the backs of your feet, towards the heels. Now settle your weight somewhere between those two points.

Shift your weight to the outsides of your feet. Shift your weight to the insides of your feet. Now settle your weight somewhere between these two points.

Feel your feet pressing into the floor. Reach the crown of your head up towards the ceiling.

Inhale your arms up to shoulder level. When they're at shoulder level, turn the palms to face up. Now bring the arms all the way up, so they're parallel to each other and to your ears. If that creates tension in the shoulders, allow the arms to be a little wider apart, more in a V-shape. See Figure 0.3 *in the Introduction for this arm position.*

Reach the fingertips up towards the ceiling, and relax the shoulders. Take three long deep breaths here. With each inhale, reach the fingertips towards the ceiling. With each exhale, relax the shoulders.

Now take five long deep breaths as you bring the arms all the way back down to your sides. The breaths can be at your own pace – just make sure that you spend at least two seconds on each inhale and two seconds on each exhale, and that the inhale and the exhale are equally long.

Check in with the client, *"What is one word that describes how your body is feeling right now?"*

As you guide the client into the pose, you will be doing it with her at the start. If your client is new to yoga, you may stand in front of her and mirror her. If she is not, you may stand to one side. Check with your client about where she would prefer that you stand, explaining to her that wherever you are, your priority is scanning her face for emotional signals, not assessing her physical form. If you are a yoga instructor, you may be used to coming behind your client to provide assists such as guiding the shoulders to relax. Notice that your being behind a client with a trauma history can be highly unnerving for her, and consider that your focus is not form, but inner experience. If you have to come behind a client for any reason, err on the side of caution and announce it and the reason for it: "I'm just going to come behind you for a moment to get a tissue."

When you check in at the end of the pose, this will be the first of many, many times that you will do so, so it is important to set the tone appropriately. Remember, you are looking for one word describing the *physical* sensation in the present moment. If you are a psychotherapist who is used to hearing your client's story in other contexts in your session, you want to gently guide your client here towards a response that is short and sweet. If the client uses two or three words – something along the lines of "warm and tingly," for example – that is fine, as long as they are still about physical sensation.

Remember also that the word is a description of the physical sensation, not an evaluation of it. So if your client answers, "ok," "good," "fine," "weird," or anything along the lines, inquire: "What are you noticing in your body?" Once they answer that, then you can rephrase the original question, "If you were to use one word to describe how you're feeling in your body, what's the first word that comes to mind?"

There are a few other words about which I like to get clarification, and these are the descriptors "light," "heavy," "hot," and "cold." I have found that different people tend to use them quite distinctly. Personally, I think of "light" as positive and "heavy" as negative. However, I have had clients for whom "light" indicates a lack of grounding, and "heavy" indicates stability. Similarly, "hot" can be a soothing warmth, or a signal that the body is overwhelmed. "Cool" can be comforting, or an indication of a shutdown. These are important distinctions for me to know, and so when I hear words the significance of which I am unsure of, I will ask something along the lines of "Tell me more about 'light,'" in order to gain a fuller understanding.

Building Self-Reliance

Focusing on the client's experience begins the process of self-reliance. The therapist provides suggestions, but ultimately, it is the client who knows the most about herself. Explaining this to the client at the outset is important, but applying it is what begins the road to healing. Scott Laurence (2010) points out that outcome-based therapy

> is guided by the client's assessments of outcomes, such as symptoms and positive change, as well as the client's assessments of the methods used and the practitioner's effectiveness. From this point of view, the consumer of the services, working closely with the therapist, is the final arbiter of whether or not the therapy is working.
>
> (p. 66)

If your client reports discomfort in a practice, ask, "If you could get more comfortable, how might you do that right now?" If he is unsure, you may provide suggestions – along the lines of "What do you gain by doing something this way versus that way?" – but let her find her comfort level (or lack thereof). Resist "fixing" things, and be open to exploration.

Assists

Many therapists who work with trauma survivors refrain from giving physical assists, as they can be triggering. As Trauma Sensitive Yoga founder David Emerson powerfully states, "No hands-on touching to assist people. We learned very clearly how destructive it was" (Emerson & Kelly, 2016, p. 83). Personally, I tend to stay away from hands-on assists when working with emotional health in general, as they are harmful at worst, and irrelevant at best. Rather than a physical goal, where a deeper stretch might aid with building flexibility or supporting alignment, here developing and connecting with an internal felt experience is paramount. An assist suggests "Here's a way of making this pose better for you," which is anathema to what we are emphasizing.

Your Countertransference

Transference refers to the redirection by the client to the therapist of emotions that were originally felt in childhood towards someone else, often a parent. Countertransference is the emotional reaction of the therapist to the client. Countertransference involves *emotions*; it goes beyond your client reminding you of your old boss, for instance. It is that your client is bringing up the same emotions in you that your boss did. You can see how this is not helpful. Even if your feeling towards your boss was positive, you are still not approaching your client with beginner's mind, and therefore not really seeing him at all. And if the thought of your old boss makes you see red, then we can *really* grasp how this does not serve your client.

Keeping track of countertransference is the ultimate practice of *yamas* and *niyamas*. Be honest with yourself and your client, and notice if you have disproportionate reactions – one way or another – towards him or her. Our minds are excellent at building complex stories, so it may take a while to realize why a particular client's mannerisms get under your skin. If you observe countertransference, seek your own healing and consultation with someone more experienced than you, in order to assess how to move forward.

Countertransference can also show up as part of your agenda. You may wish to address something in a client because it may be an aspect you inadvertently hope to heal in yourself or in someone in your life. But that may not be something that is on your client's agenda. Again, be honest, and seek your own healing.

Takeaway

At the end of the session, it is helpful to note the takeaway. "What's one thing you got out of today?" you may inquire of your client. There is value especially in having a takeaway that your client can incorporate into his daily routine. After the intake session, that takeaway would be a grounding practice, whether Mountain pose or a breath with the same number of inhales and exhales, such as the breath we used while we were lowering the arms in Mountain. The easier the practice, the more likely the client will be to turn to it.

While the takeaway is a helpful tool, it is important also to note that using it is not an imperative element on the path to healing. As Rhodes (2015) points out in her study on yoga for trauma,

> Although maintenance of practice was identified by participants as an important dimension of sustaining and increasing the benefits derived from yoga, few had practices that were more frequent than one time per week. This indicates that significant gains could be made without a large time commitment.
>
> (p. 255)

Streeter et al.'s study (2017) showed no significant difference in symptom reduction between those who practiced yoga three times a week and those who did so twice. Therefore, we will discuss the takeaway only in certain instances where it is especially valuable (Chapters 7 and 8). But know that it is always an option for any client at any point.

Moving Forward

In the next chapters, we will learn how to build a therapeutic practice. As we move through, allow time to assess the effects of each piece that you add. Remember that this is not about building physical but emotional conditioning, which means being in the moment rather than distracting ourselves. Adding more parts rapidly is a way of distracting the mind away from the physical sensations.

Instead, we are focusing on what in Somatic Experiencing is referred to as "titration," which means processing activation in bite-sized pieces. If you find yourself eager to move fast either due to client pressure or other stories you may be telling yourself ("the client must be getting bored"), bring to mind and, if relevant, share this analogy with your client: just as we do not eat a sandwich in one gulp but in bite-sized, well-chewed pieces, so it is with emotional processing. We allow effects to unfold before adding practices. We do not want to keep taking more and more bites when we have not chewed what we have in our mouths.

When you evaluate pacing, note not just what the client is telling you, but also what she is showing you. Be aware of shifts outside of the client's window of affect tolerance, which means signs that the client has become overwhelmed and is now hyper- or hypoaroused. While hyperarousal can manifest as emotional expression and hypoarousal as emotional shutdown, most people's discomfort will become apparent via more minor signs, such as fidgeting or other psychomotor agitation, or shifts in eye contact, voice, or breathing patterns.

When You're Not the Right Fit

In an ideal world, your client comes in, works with you, and starts to feel better. As he improves, you begin discussing decreasing the regularity of your sessions, eventually titrating down to termination, with the understanding that the door is always open for the client to return. But that is not what always happens. Sometimes, a few sessions in, you realize that you are not the correct fit for this client. You find that his needs are outside your scope of competence.

In any scenario, it is always appropriate to check in with your client every so often to see if therapy is working for him, or whether he would like something to be different. In most cases, a check-in like that will help you identify and clarify any mismatches. But if your client's needs are outside your scope, no amount of checking in will alter that. Ask yourself: if I received a few hours of additional training or consultation with someone who is more experienced, would that be enough to change things? If the answer is "no," then it is appropriate for you to let the client know that you have come to realize that his needs are outside of your scope, and provide him with appropriate referrals. You may be tempted to keep pushing through, but do not hold on to a situation where you are clearly not serving your client because you are too uncomfortable to have a conversation about it.

Taking Care of Yourself

As you start working with clients, be careful to maintain your own self-care. Therapist burnout, also referred to as secondary/vicarious trauma or compassion fatigue, is a common challenge (cf. Wu, 2015), and it can seriously hinder therapists' work if unaddressed. Inadequate self-care and subsequent burnout can lead to loss of empathy, inattention, impatience, irritability, or unrecognized countertransference (Gerbarg & Brown, 2015).

Becoming aware of the signs of burnout is the first step. The following are some red flags:

- Preoccupation with the traumatic stories of the people you work with. You want to be present for clients in the moment, but not take the feelings home.
- Emotional symptoms of anger, grief, mood swings, anxiety, or depression.
- Physical issues related to stress, such as headaches, stomach aches, fatigue, or problems sleeping.
- Feeling burned out, powerless, hopeless, disillusioned, irritable, and/ or angry towards "the system."
- A tendency to self-isolate, be tardy, avoid certain people, or experience a lack of empathy and loss of motivation.

Developing a self-care strategy is key to preventing or overcoming burnout:

- *Maintain a work–life balance.* This involves taking time off to recharge and avoiding working long hours and/or carrying too heavy a caseload or workload. It is important to figure out what is an appropriate caseload for you, and what your tipping point is. Your appropriate caseload may end up being lower than the total number of hours you need to or can work, in which case you may need to supplement your caseload with something else (e.g. general population yoga classes if you are a yoga therapist).
- *Figure out a way to release your load at the end of the day.* Every day before leaving my office, I sit for a moment and bring to mind the clients I saw that day. Then I envision releasing them with love and light towards their journey of healing. If there something on which I need to follow up before I next see them, I set an intention to follow up on that piece without my ego taking on emotions or energy that are not necessary for the task.
- *Maintain your yoga practice.* One of the ironic developments that may occur is that as we guide others towards yoga, we step away from our own practice because we "don't have time" for it. Investing the time will provide a return in spades, as you well know from your previous experiences with yoga.
- *Develop a good social network.* Having a good support system in place is crucial in order to be able to connect with others in a meaningful way. It also helps you maintain appropriate boundaries with your clients so that you do not end up relying on them for social support.

- *Reconnect with nature.* Being out in nature is therapeutic, whether you go for a hike in the woods, or a walk on the beach, or just do a little gardening.
- *Get involved with activities outside of work.* Take your mind off work by taking a class or engaging in a creative endeavor such as drawing, painting, or writing.
- *Seek your own healing.* Figure out what helps you heal. Personally, one thing I do is schedule a massage every two weeks. And never hesitate to seek your own therapy.

Intake Questions for Emotional Health

1 Please list the healthcare practitioners with whom you are currently working. Include physicians, psychotherapists, and any practitioners of Complementary/ Alternative Medicine.

Name:	Name:	Name:
Specialization:	Specialization:	Specialization:
Address:	Address:	Address:
Office phone:	Office phone:	Office phone:
Email:	Email:	Email:

2 Does your doctor/healthcare practitioner know that you are participating in Yoga Therapy?
Y N

3 Collaboration among healthcare providers can lead to a more thorough approach to your care. Do we have your permission, if needed, to contact other members of your healthcare team?
Y N
If you answered yes to the above question, kindly complete an information disclosure form.

4 List any diagnoses you have been given, and treatment options followed to date:

Diagnosis:	Diagnosis:	Diagnosis:
Date of diagnosis:	Date of diagnosis:	Date of diagnosis:
Who made it:	Who made it:	Who made it:
Any family history of diagnosis:	Any family history of diagnosis:	Any family history diagnosis:
Symptoms present:	Symptoms present:	Symptoms present:
Treatment(s) attempted:	Treatment(s) attempted:	Treatment(s) attempted:
Success of treatment:	Success of treatment:	Success of treatment:

5 List your medication history (over-the-counter and prescription). Include any vitamins, minerals, tinctures, and herbal supplements.

Medication:	Medication:	Medication:
Dosage:	Dosage:	Dosage:
Frequency:	Frequency:	Frequency:
Length of time:	Length of time:	Length of time:
Reason for taking:	Reason for taking:	Reason for taking:
Effects and side effects:	Effects and side effects:	Effects and side effects:

6 What are your primary reasons for coming in for Yoga Therapy?
   a.
   b.
   c.

7 Do you currently practice yoga? Y N
   If yes:
   a. How often and which style?
   b. Where do you practice?
   c. What aspects of your practice do you find most helpful for your emotional health?
   d. What is your favorite pose and/or breath, and why?

8 Are there currently aspects of your life that give you joy and pleasure? Y N
   If yes, what are they?

9 Do you have a creative outlet (e.g., singing, journaling, writing, dancing, art, gardening, crafts projects, etc.?) Y N
   If yes, what is it? How frequently do you turn to it?

10 What are some sources of support for you? May I contact them in case of an emergency? If yes, please provide their contact information.

References

Douglass, L. (2011). Thinking through the body: The conceptualization of yoga as therapy for individuals with eating disorders. *Eating Disorders, 19*(1), 83–96. doi: 10.1080/10640266.2011.533607

Elgelid, S. (2015). Yoga, is it learning or therapy? Comparing medical and educational models. In E. G. Horovitz & S. Elgelid (Eds.), *Yoga therapy: Theory and practice* (pp. 119–130). New York & London: Routledge.

Emerson, D. (2015). *Trauma-sensitive yoga in therapy: Bringing the body into treatment.* New York & London: W. W. Norton & Company.

Emerson, D., & Kelly, J. (2016). Yoga as an adjunctive treatment for posttraumatic stress disorder: A conversation with David Emerson. In C. Costin & J. Kelly

(Eds.), *Yoga and eating disorders: Ancient healing for modern illness* (pp. 79–85). New York, NY: Routledge.

Gerbarg, P. L., & Brown, R. P. (2015). Yoga and neuronal pathways to enhance stress response: Emotion regulation, bonding, and spirituality. In E. G. Horovitz & S. Elgelid (Eds.), *Yoga therapy: Theory and practice* (pp. 61–75). New York & London: Routledge.

Horovitz, E. G. (2015). Appendices. In E. G. Horovitz & S. Elgelid (Eds.), *Yoga therapy: Theory and practice* (pp. 61–75). New York & London: Routledge.

International Association of Yoga Therapists (2016, September 1). Scope of practice for yoga therapy. Retrieved April 7, 2018 from International Association of Yoga Therapists: http://c.ymcdn.com/sites/www.iayt.org/resource/resmgr/docs_ Certification_ALL/docs_certification/scopeofpractice/2016-09-01_iayt_scope_ of_pra.pdf

Laurence, S. (2010). Issues in yoga therapy: The role of outcome-based standards in yoga therapy. *International Journal of Yoga Therapy, 20*(1), 65–71. Retrieved 21 June, 2018 from https://yogafordepression.com/wp-content/uploads/the-role-of-outcome-based-standards-in-yoga-therapy-scott-laurence.pdf

Lilly, M., & Hedlund, J. (2010). Yoga therapy in practice: Healing childhood sexual abuse with yoga. *International Journal of Yoga Therapy, 20,* 120–130. sRetrieved from https://yogafordepression.com/wp-content/uploads/healing-childhood-sexual-abuse-with-yoga-lilly-and-hedlund.pdf

Rhodes, A. (2015). Claiming peaceful embodiment through yoga in the aftermath of trauma. *Complementary Therapies in Clinical Practice, 21*(4), 247–256. doi: 10.1016/j.ctcp.2015.09.004

Rizopoulos, N. (2017, November). Practice well: Embodying the Sutra. *Yoga Journal*, p. 52.

Streeter, C. C., Gerbarg, P. L., Whitfield, T. H., Owen, L., Johnston, J., Silveri, M. M., … Jensen, J. E. (2017). Treatment of major depressive disorder with Iyengar yoga and coherent breathing: A randomized controlled dosing study. *Journal of Alternative and Complementary Medicine, 23*(3), 201–207. doi: 10.1089/ acm.2016.0140

van der Kolk, B. A. (2015). *The body keeps the score: Brain, mind, and body in the healing of trauma*. New York, NY: Penguin Books.

Visceglia, E. (2015). Psychiatry and yoga therapy. In L. Payne, T. Gold, E. Goldman, & C. Rosenberg (Eds.), *Yoga therapy & integrative medicine: Where ancient science meets modern medicine* (pp. 143–155). Laguna Beach, CA: Basic Health Publications.

Wu, J. (2015). Yoga therapy for our healers: How to give to self to give to others. In E. G. Horovitz & S. Elgelid (Eds.), *Yoga therapy: Theory and practice* (pp. 103–118). New York & London: Routledge.

5 Grounding and Creating Presence

You have met with your client, found out more about him via your assessment, explored exteroception and interoception, and introduced grounding. This chapter picks up from there, focusing more on grounding, stabilizing poses. Whether you are working with a client or on yourself, this is always the starting point. This is the category of practices with which to stay in two other instances: 1) for any imbalance where there is a loss of contact with reality (e.g., psychosis, trauma disorders, or personality disorders), and 2) for co-occurring dulling (*mudha*) and agitation (*ksipta*) symptoms (e.g., bipolar disorder, or comorbid anxiety and depression).

One of the challenges of emotional imbalance is that our minds are focusing on something that happened in the past or that might happen in the future. Regardless of whether our thoughts are chattering and spinning, jumping from one thing or another, or fixated in seeming slow motion on the memory or anticipation of a single element, the challenge of being somewhere in the past or the future is that the thoughts and emotions that we are experiencing are not related to something that is actually real. Our mind thinks it is real, but it is just an aspect of a representation that happened or might happen, rather than what is happening now.

For example, let us say that I was in a serious car accident, and find myself – understandably – thinking about it all the time. I replay it in my mind, and as I replay it, I find my anxiety rising, I am breaking out in a sweat, and I am beginning to feel a panic. My body is acting as if I were in the car accident right now. But I am not. I am at home in my PJs, and it is the power of my mind that is leading the rest of my body to act as if I were still experiencing the car accident.

So how do I use my body to remind myself that I am not in a car accident right now, but rather, at home in my PJs? Maybe I look around, and focus on everything I am observing. Maybe I touch my PJs – which I would definitely not be wearing outside – and notice their fabric. Perhaps I press my feet into the floor, and notice that contact. And now, I notice my physical sensations, such as the butterflies in my stomach, the tightening of my chest, and the sweating, and recognize them as sensations. By using a balance of exteroception and interoception, I am slowly giving my mind something to focus on other than the images of the traumatic event.

Depending on the intensity of the symptoms a person feels, the length of time they have had them, and what other connections they relate to in their mind, practices such as these may or may not bring relief. For some, they will. But sometimes, the feeling of trauma is so strong that we cannot even sense these distinct feelings and their physical manifestations. We are constantly triggered, either at the height of emotion or frozen, so we need a consistent practice of returning to the present before we can really believe that the thoughts and emotions we are having are not directly related to the immediate moment.

You can see here why it is, therefore, crucial that you make sure that your client is completely grounded before trying to work more directly with raising or calming energy and, therefore, emotions. If I am not fully in the present, then an effort to raise my energy can just lead me to let loose further emotion that I may be unable to contain, and that will unsettle me even more. I first learned this the hard way when I introduced the breath of joy to someone experiencing depression. I thought that it would lift her spirits and her mood, and instead it ended up unleashing lengthy, deep waves of emotion. Sometimes we move emotion and it is a release, a catharsis, and we feel better. Other times we end up mired in that sadness, and that was what happened for her. It was in my fumbling for how to help that I came upon the thought that she needed to be grounded back into the present moment. Then I saw the sobs subside, the chest shift to fuller breathing, and the shoulders relax. She was now here.

Bessel van der Kolk describes a similar experience. "In our first yoga study," he details,

> we had a 50 percent dropout rate, the highest of any study we'd ever done. When we interviewed the patients who'd left, we learned that they had found the program too intense: Any posture that involved the pelvis could precipitate intense panic or even flashbacks to sexual assaults. Intense physical sensations unleashed the demons from the past that had been so carefully kept in check by numbing and inattention. This taught us to go slow, often at a snail's pace. That approach paid off: In our most recent study only one of thirty-four participants did not finish.

(2015, p. 276)

For those of us who are therapists, we can become addicted to practices that elicit tears. For yoga therapists, it can be tempting to place someone who we know is experiencing depression into a "heart opening" pose. But as we discussed in the previous chapter, the most important gift of yoga is a practice that is in the here and now.

Asking someone if they are in the present is not enough – we may think we are when we are not. It takes going through a grounding practice fully and repeatedly to really be able to assess whether someone experiencing emotional imbalance now feels stable enough to begin working on shifting energetically. Grounding practices serve as an excellent bridge to mindfulness: the mental state achieved by focusing one's awareness on the present moment, while acknowledging and accepting one's feelings, thoughts, and bodily sensations.

Who Benefits from Grounding?

Everyone! A grounding practice does several things:

- Builds a sense of centeredness and empowerment
- Allows gradual, safer progression
- Provides a context for a group practice with clients who have differing emotional health imbalances or are at different points on their journeys.

As mentioned earlier, there are two general instances when you would focus someone's entire practice on grounding without envisioning a shift into *brahmana* or *langhana*. The first is when they are not rooted in the present in general. This includes diagnoses that involve dissociation, such as posttraumatic stress disorder (PTSD); the potential for hallucinations, such as schizophrenia and bipolar disorder; or an uneven way of viewing the world, such as personality disorders. For example, people with schizophrenia have been found to have a heightened baseline level of physiological arousal – so that the body is chronically agitated even under normal conditions – while the parasympathetic nervous system, the body's means of calming itself, is underactive (Visceglia, 2015). While this may lead us to believe that a *langhana* practice may be more appropriate, in fact, in vulnerable individuals, mania and psychotic episodes have occurred as a result of meditation even in individuals without a history of psychosis (da Silva, Ravindran, & Ravindran, 2009, p. 13). The slowing down and focusing inwards in those instances may be overwhelming emotionally, leading to the loosening of cognitive controls.

The second instance is when a client has symptoms that provide a mix of agitation and dullness. This includes diagnoses in which the two can be sequential, such as bipolar disorder or cyclothymia, as well as simultaneous, such as co-occurring anxiety and depression. In Chapter 2, we mentioned the study (Uebelacker, Weinstock, & Kraines, 2014) in which five respondents with bipolar disorder gave specific examples of times they believed a yoga practice had led to increased agitation, and five gave specific examples of times that they believed a yoga practice had led to increased depression or lethargy. It is, therefore, crucial to pay attention to creating stability for participants, rather than being pulled to try treating one set of symptoms or another.

What Does Grounding Entail?

A grounding practice typically involves the following:

- Poses where contact with the floor is emphasized.
- Poses that are symmetrical, where both sides of the body (if physically available) are making equal contact with the floor.
- Poses where the body is composed mainly of straight lines (i.e., no twists).
- Poses where the torso is upright (i.e., no forward or back bending).
- Breaths with equal length inhales and exhales.
- Visualizations of feeling stable and rooted.
- Constant check-in with physical sensations.
- Active engagement. At all times, the client is focused on something, whether it is activating a part of the body or synchronizing movement with breath in some manner.
- Having the eyes open, to focus on the here and now.
- A morning practice, in order to set the tone for the day. However, it is deeply beneficial to return to grounding at any time of day.

Beginning the Practice

Orienting to the Space

The first step to being present is orienting to the space. To return to the example of the car accident at the start of this chapter, when my mind really accepts that I am safe in my home or my therapist's office, not in the car where the accident occurred, it can let go of some of the thoughts associated with the trauma and the related symptoms of anxiety. There are two seated techniques that I tend to use to orient to the space, both of which we saw in Chapter 4. Again, here and throughout this and subsequent chapters, whatever is in italics is what I would say out loud to guide the client.

54321 Grounding Technique

> *Look around the room. Say out loud:*

- *5 things that you see*
- *4 things that you're touching, or are touching you*
- *3 things that you hear*
- *2 things that you smell*
- *1 taste in your mouth*

When I do this with an individual client, I guide him to answer out loud, so it is easy to know when to move on to the next category. If I am doing this with a group, I guide them to do it in silence so that they can come up with their own responses undistracted. In either case, I allow the pause between each category and the next to be a little longer each time. This is for two reasons. First, the responses to each category (except for the last one) are a little harder to discern than the previous one, so more time is needed. Second, as the client becomes comfortable, slowing my pace will allow him to relax a little more, whereas a slower start may feel too abrupt at the outset of the session.

Looking at an Object

> *Now look around the room, and allow your eye to land on something that pleases you.*
> *Notice what it is in your body that indicates to you that it pleases you.*

As mentioned in Chapter 4, I use this exercise for several reasons. First, it allows the client to find something pleasant (if that turns out to be too difficult, then here I alter the cue to finding something neutral). Second, it allows him to notice physical cues of ease, not just of difficulty. Third, it serves as a bridge between focus on the external environment and on internal physical sensations, to which I am about to go next.

Orienting to the Body

Now gazing at a point on the floor in front of you, notice how your body feels. Starting at the tips of your toes, move slowly up your legs, into your torso, up to your shoulders, to your neck, to your head, and notice how you feel. Notice areas that stand out in your body, and areas that feel neutral.

Now press your feet into the floor, and notice the contact between your feet and the floor. Press your legs into the chair, and notice the contact between your legs and the chair. Notice the contact/distance between your back and the back of the chair.

Reach the crown of the head up towards the ceiling, and relax the shoulders. Now take a breath in, and reach the crown of the head up towards the ceiling. Take a breath out, and relax the shoulders. Again, take a breath in, and reach the crown up, and a breath out, and relax the shoulders. Do it twice more at your own pace.

My goal is to do all three portions with a client, but at the start, I might just do one of these if I notice that it is difficult for the client to keep her attention on the practice. Note that throughout, I have given the client something active to do. I am alerting her directly to be aware of a specific part of the body (e.g., the body scan in the first segment), to activate a particular part of the body (e.g., pressing the feet/legs in the second segment), or to synchronize breath and movement (e.g., inhaling and reaching the crown of the head up, then exhaling and relaxing the shoulders, in the third segment). For each segment, I want to allow a couple of seconds for the client to engage and notice, without letting the silence become so long that she loses the grounding and her mind goes elsewhere.

Throughout, I am watching for signs of engagement and/or dissociation, especially via the gaze or the breath, allowing me to gather information on how long a pause time is appropriate for my client. Remember, if your client is inclined towards dissociation, if you do not give them something to do, they will check out and be elsewhere, even as they follow your cues. But do not err on the side of overdoing and giving the client a ton of cues to follow just a simple physical movement on the inhale and another on the exhale can be sufficient.

Warm-Ups

Warm-ups serve two main functions. The primary one is straightforward: to generate some heat in the body. But they are also the first time that the client will move his body beyond a straightforward seated position, so they serve as the earliest opportunity for the clinician to see what movement might elicit.

While warm-ups can be done in a chair, I tend to limit seated warm-ups unless this is the only option physically available to a client. Poses where the body is making contact with the floor are far more effective in serving as a grounding tool. Furthermore, moving the body to a less familiar position can help bring the mind more into the present.

Again, the more engaging the warm-up, the more it helps the client remain present in the moment. That does not mean that it should be challenging physically, but rather, that it should absorb the mind in the moment. In fact, a pose that is challenging physically can bring about a great deal of mind chatter connecting to fear, ineptitude, and failure, thereby pushing the client out of the moment and into her head once more.

The Universal Warm-Up

One of my favorite ways to warm up is via a sequence that I have put together that I refer to as "the universal warm-up." I call it this because I do it with almost all clients for whom it is physically viable. In it, the body is always in straight lines, there is strong contact between the body and the floor, and all poses are symmetrical.

Starting at the back of the space, sit on your heels.

Inhale and come up on your knees. Reach the arms up, and notice them reaching towards the ceiling.

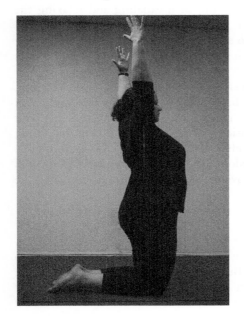

Figure 5.1

Exhale, and hinge forward into a puppy stretch.

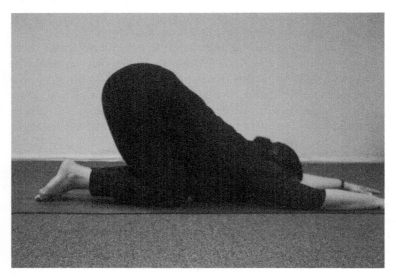

Figure 5.2

Inhale, and come to all fours. Make sure that the hands are underneath the shoulders, knees are underneath the hips. Spread the fingers wide, and press the fingers into the floor. Notice the contact between the fingers and the floor.

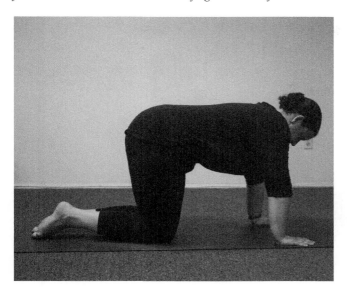

Figure 5.3

Exhale, rounding the spine, coming into a cat stretch.

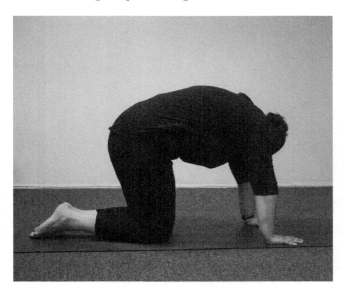

Figure 5.4

Inhale, pressing the hands into the floor. Bring the tailbone up, drop the belly down, bring the shoulders back, and look straight ahead of you, coming into cow pose.

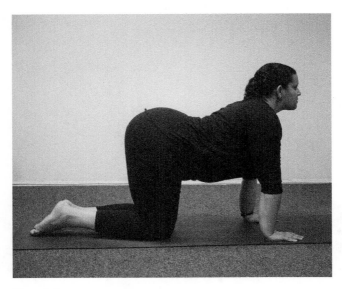

Figure 5.5

Exhale, tuck the toes under, coming into downward-facing dog. Let the knees be as straight or as bent as works for you. Continue to press into the fingers, slide the shoulders away from the ears, and relax your neck, so that the head is hanging loose.

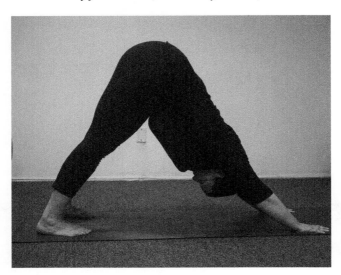

Figure 5.6

Inhale, coming back onto all fours.

Exhale, come to sit back on your heels.

Check in with your client, asking, *"What is one word that describes how your body feels right now?"*

If appropriate, repeat the sequence twice more.

What to Notice

As your client is moving, notice his breath. Is he actually inhaling and exhaling throughout? If not, gently guide him to become aware of his breath. For our purposes here, the client and you do not need to get tangled up in when the inhale and when the exhale occur, as long as you see that he is not holding his breath.

The verbal check-in is a central part of your work. Doing it is vital, and how you do it is also important. You may wish to spend some time reminding the client of the nature of the check-in before you engage in any actual *asanas* or *pranayamas*. Explain to your client that you are inviting her to notice her body, not the story in her mind. Therefore, you are inviting her to come up with a word that describes how her *body* feels in the moment. The invitation is not "How are you feeling now?" which can definitely elicit a story related to another time ("I feel ok, but I still don't understand why he did that") or even "What is one word that describes how you're feeling right now?" ("Confused"). The focus is on the body, and the present moment: "What is one word that describes how your *body* feels *right now?*"

Remind your client that any word or phrase that she comes up with is appropriate, and that she should say the first thing that comes to mind *after* the pose, rather than spend time thinking about it during the pose. It is fine if she is repeating a word from one pose to the next, as long as it describes how she really feels in that precise moment.

Once the client says the word, repeat it back. Regardless of what the word is, repeat it in the same tone of voice, signaling your openness to whatever experience the client is having. Resist adding a positive judgment if the word is positive, or a reactive intention to shift things if it is negative. So, if the client says, "Calm," repeat back, "Calm" rather than "Calm. Good." The latter signals that you would prefer to hear something positive, and it potentially shuts down your client's report of a more challenging emotion.

Especially important is what you do with a word that suggests a more challenging emotion. Allowing space for it is one of the most significant ways that you can be present for your client. Your client has probably received signals from others in the past that there is no room for his symptoms of depression, anxiety, or whatever else he might be experiencing. Others may have told him to "get over it," "move on," or "think positive," or they may have had manifold quick fix suggestions: "You should go for a walk," or "You should meditate." Often we do not encourage challenging emotions in others because we do not know how to be with them. Allowing your client to have them can be quite liberating, and once your client feels them – the real feelings in the present, not the mind chatter and story around them – that can open the way to move with and maybe through them.

So if you ask your client for the one word that describes how their body feels right now, and they say, "Agitated," simply repeat that as you would any other word. Resist adding, "Well, let's see if we can shift that," or "Let's do something else that will help you feel better." Allow the emotion to be there, and allow the next step to be in the client's hands. Ask, "Would you like to go through this sequence again, or would you prefer to do something else?" Sometimes the second time feels different for the client, and neither you nor they will know whether it will unless they try it. But also, there is no need to force them to try it: they are the best judge of their window of affect tolerance.

Also, resist connecting the question with their response: "Since this made you feel agitated, would you like to go through this sequence again, or would you prefer to do something else?" That still implicitly marks their response as problematic, rather than as one possibility among many. Your own practice of witness consciousness and non-attachment to outcome can work wonders for the client.

The variety of possible responses highlights the importance of your approaching any practice with non-attachment to outcome. If you label a practice, "Now we're going to do something relaxing" or "Now we're going to come into a nice stretch," that dictates outcome. If I, as the client, end up feeling not so relaxed or nice at the end of it, I may think that I did something wrong, and that may connect with a general story of "I always do everything wrong." Or I may end up thinking that this sequence is relaxing for everyone except me, so there really must be something wrong with me.

As I mentioned in Chapter 4, there are a few one-word responses for which I tend to ask for more clarification. The first category is that of evaluations, such as "good," "nice," or "ok." These do not really describe a physical sensation. Does "good" mean grounded/stable or excited? And is the emphasis in "ok" that the client does not feel great, or that she does not feel terrible? The second category is regarding the words "light," "heavy," "hot," and "cold.". When I receive one of these responses, I prompt, "Tell me more about 'cold.'" That usually elicits another word or two that clarifies things.

It is important for the response to be brief, in order to keep the person in the body and therefore the present. Sometimes your client may answer the question and then start talking about something else. Listen a little, and then gently guide him back to the body, explaining that the challenge here for both of you is to remain in the body, as tempting as it might be to move into the story and have a more typical conversation.

Building the Practice: *Asanas*

Types of Standing Poses

An obvious place to start with grounding is standing poses. After all, the feet are on the ground, which should make these poses grounding, right? But, in fact, we can group standing poses into four categories:

Poses Emphasizing Solidity

This is the category of poses we will use for grounding. They include Mountain (*Tadasana*), Standing Squat (*Utkatasana*), Warrior II (*Virabhadrasana* II), and even a version of Side Angle (*Parsvakonasana*).

Poses Emphasizing Heat

This category includes poses that have a more solid base, but also a side-to-side movement, slight backbend in the torso, and/or a deeper opening in the hips. These movements generally serve to heat the body. We will encounter some of them in the next chapter, for our *brahmana* practice. They include: Half Moon (*Ardha Chandrasana*), Goddess (*Utkata Konasana*), Triangle (*Trikonasana*), Crescent (*Anjaneyasana*), Warrior I (*Virabhadrasana* I), Reverse Warrior (*Viparita Virabhadrasana*), Revolved Triangle (*Parivrtta Trikonasana*), and Revolved Side Angle (*Parivrtta Parsvakonasana*).

Poses Emphasizing Release

This category involves forward bends, which lead to release, thereby cooling the body and calming the mind. We will address a couple of these in Chapter 7 for our *langhana* practice, although Pyramid is interspersed among other poses in our *brahmana* practice. They include: Pyramid (*Parsvottanasana*), Standing Fold (*Uttanasana*), and Wide-Legged Forward Bend (*Prasarita Padottanasana*).

Poses Emphasizing Balance

These include Balancing Half Moon (*Ardha Chandrasana*), Tree (*Vriksasana*), Eagle (*Garudasana*), Dancer (*Natarajasana*), and Extended Hand to Big Toe Pose (*Utthita Hasta Padangustasana*). Since balance in the body varies from day to day and often has evaluative chatter of success or failure attached to it, and since people often hold their breath during balance poses, thereby increasing agitation, we will generally stay away from this category. One exception is that we will incorporate a balance pose in our work with attention deficit hyperactivity disorder (ADHD), which we will discuss in Chapter 7.

Another instance in which we will turn to a balance pose is if a client specifically mentions – at intake or later – that one from an existing practice helps them feels grounded, energized, or calmed. For instance, when I asked one of my clients today which pose from her yoga practice at her studio helped her feel stable, she immediately said, "Dancer pose," as no matter how much she wobbles in it, she still feels solid in her core. That is a very helpful analogy (inner stability amidst outside turmoil), and therefore, we will return to it and Dancer pose again.

Standing Poses Category 1 – Poses Emphasizing Solidity

Mountain

In Chapter 4 we introduced Mountain, a basic standing pose, with language that emphasized grounding and engagement. Mountain is a pose that you can keep repeating with your client at the start of each practice, potentially lengthening its hold with time. See Chapter 4 for the words with which to guide your client in and out of the pose.

If your client experiences challenging emotions in Mountain, they may well not be ready to progress to something else. Stay with Mountain until your client arrives at a point when they are generally able to access some sense of grounding/stability in it. That does not mean that you will keep repeating it in the one session, but rather, that you may practice it a few times, interspersed with some *pranayama* or *mantra* meditation (see later). In general, you want your client to access grounding/stability consistently in a pose before you add another. Familiarity lowers anxiety and builds a sense of safety.

Once your client consistently feels grounding/stability in Mountain – whether that happens the first few times you practice it or over the course of many sessions – you can now add another grounding pose. And if standing Mountain is not appropriate for your client, you can do it in a chair, still pressing the feet into the ground and lifting the arms up if viable. Or you can do Staff pose instead.

Staff

Sit on the floor with legs extended. There is a straight line between the middle of the knee and the second toe.

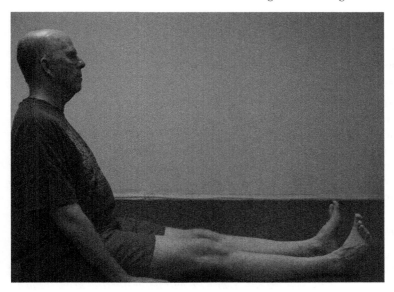

Figure 5.7

If needed, rest the back against the wall, and/or place a rolled blanket underneath the knees for hamstring support.

To add to the pose, bring the arms up so that they are parallel to the ears, as you would for Mountain. Inhale, reach the fingertips up towards the ceiling.

Exhale, maintain that length in the arms, and relax the shoulders.

Inhale, feel the contact between the buttocks and the floor. Exhale, relax the shoulders. Repeat three more times.

Slowly release the arms down by your sides.

Check in with your client, asking, *"What is one word that describes how your body feels right now?"*

Because of its seated nature, Staff pose tends to be less grounding than Mountain. It is far easier for the average person to become distracted while seated than while standing, so do not spend too much time in this pose at the expense of a standing pose, unless you are working with someone for whom standing poses are a challenge. However, if sitting requires physical effort for your client, that will help make the pose more grounding.

Standing Squat

Once your client feels consistently grounded/stable in Mountain pose, you can introduce a standing squat.

Stand with your feet hip-width apart. Raise your arms up to shoulder level, palms down.

Bend at the knees, and sit back as if you're sitting in a chair. Make sure that your knees don't go past your toes.

Straighten the legs, and slowly release the arms down by your sides.

Check in with your client, asking, *"What is one word that describes how your body feels right now?"*

Standing squat is a grounding pose that can also be energizing, so when you introduce it, only do it once, even if your client reports a positive experience. If your client returns the next week still feeling positive, then you can try twice in a row. Always add gradually, and allow time in the middle for integration. Sometimes the effect of a pose is felt later, rather than while practicing it. Note also that the standing squat involves hip movement, which can sometimes release emotions.

Variation: Standing Squat with Back against the Wall

You can also use the wall to increase grounding and stability.

Stand with your back against the wall, arms by your sides. Bend into your knees, and as you bend, walk your feet out. Your back will naturally slide down the wall.

Continue to do so, until your knees get as close to a 90-degree bend as is comfortable for you. As you inhale, feel your feet pressing into the floor, and as you exhale, relax your shoulders.

Check in with your client, asking, *"What is one word that describes how your body feels right now?"*

Variation: Standing Squat with Raised Arms

Once you know that your client feels stable/grounded, you can move on to a more active variation of the pose, and see how this is for him.

Stand with your feet hip-width apart. Raise the arms up to shoulder level, and then all the way up so they are parallel by your ears (like they are in Mountain).

Bend at the knees, and sit back as if you're sitting in a chair. Make sure that your knees don't go past your toes.

Inhale, reach the fingertips up towards the ceiling. Exhale, maintain that length in the arms, and relax the shoulders.

Inhale, press the feet into the floor. Exhale, relax the shoulders. Repeat three more times.

Slowly straighten the legs, and release the arms down by your sides.

Check in with your client, asking, *"What is one word that describes how your body feels right now?"*

Warrior II

All the previous poses have been symmetrical. Now we will experiment with a two-sided pose that also involves movement in the hips. As usual, proceed slowly, noticing your client's verbal and non-verbal cues.

Stand with your feet hip-width apart. Step one foot out wide.

Turn your right foot out 90 degrees, and your left foot in 15–30 degrees.

Bend into your right knee. Widen your stance so that when you bend your right knee, it remains in line with your right ankle, not moving towards your toes.

Bring your left hand on your left hip, and bring the left hip back. The fronts of both hips should face the wall in front of you.

Bring the arms out at shoulder level, palms down. Turn your head to look over your right index finger.

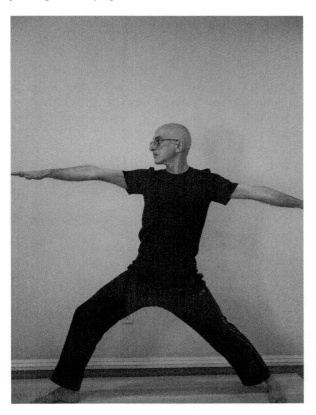

Figure 5.8

Inhale, press into your feet and reach through your fingers, spreading them wide. Exhale, and relax the shoulders. Repeat the breath and movement three times.

To release, straighten the right leg. Bring the arms down by your sides. Turn the toes of both feet forward.

Step the feet hip-width apart, arms come up by your ears (so you are back in Mountain), and release the arms down. Shake everything out.

Check in with your client, asking, "*What is one word that describes how your body feels right now?*" Get ready to repeat on the other side.

At first, you will want to guide your client to take a break between the two sides and see how that is for her. Even if your client is a seasoned yogi with the muscular strength to hold the pose, you are still looking for the grounding effect, and progressing gradually allows you to do that.

When your client feels consistently grounded in the pose, you can go straight from one side to the other, without coming out of the pose in the middle. Instead of turning both feet forward, you would guide her automatically after the first side to turn the left foot out 90 degrees and the right foot in 15–30 degrees, and proceed to the posture on the other side. Again, build both the hold time and the repetitions slowly.

Flowing between Warrior II and Side Angle

Once your client feels grounded here, you can begin experimenting with shifting the uprightness of the torso, and seeing how that affects him.

From Warrior II on the first side, inhale and bring your right forearm onto your right leg. Reach the left arm straight up towards the ceiling.

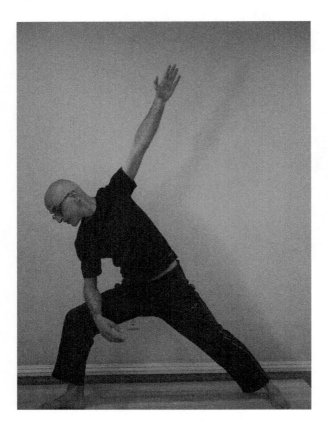

Figure 5.9

Exhale back to Warrior II, reaching through the fingertips. Repeat twice.
Transition to the other side, and do the same.

Check in with your client, asking, "*What is one word that describes how your body feels right now?*"

This flow between Warrior II and Side Angle serves to test the waters for potential progression away from grounding poses if your client is a candidate for a *brahmana* or *langhana* practice. Stay with it for a while, to make sure that your client feels grounded now that he is practicing a flow. Remain with this version of side angle with the forearm on the leg, rather than that with the hand on the floor, which creates too much of a bend in the torso for grounding. Continue to work with other grounding poses alongside this flow.

Downward-Facing Dog

You have already practiced downward-facing dog with your client during the universal warm-up, so she is familiar with it. Now you can practice focusing on more grounding.

Come to your hands and knees. Make sure that the hands are directly below the shoulders, and the knees are directly below the hips. Spread the fingers wide, with the middle finger pointing straight forward.

Press into your fingers, tuck your toes under, and lift your knees off the floor. Keep your knees bent.

Continue to feel your fingers pressing into the floor. Inhale and bend into your right knee, straightening your left leg. Exhale and bend into your left knee, straightening your right leg. Repeat two more times.

Bring the knees back to the floor, and come to sitting.

Check in with your client, asking, "*What is one word that describes how your body feels right now?*"

Do not bring your client into child's pose after this downward dog, even if you may be tempted to do so. The point is to ground your client, and child's pose is a movement that instead invites a retreat inward. If you are working with someone with emotional dysregulation or dissociation, you can lose the grounding that you gained with downward-facing dog by doing an inward-focusing pose like child.

Once your client feels grounded in downward dog, you can experiment with lengthening the hold. In that case, after inviting the client to bend and straighten alternate knees for three breaths, you can invite him for a few breaths to inhale and press into the fingers (not the palm area by the wrist, which puts pressure on the wrist joint), and exhale, relaxing the shoulders away from the ears.

Beginning and Building the
Practice: *Pranayama* and Meditation

In describing her work with yoga and emotional health, psychiatrist Elizabeth Visceglia (2015) relates her work with a 28-year-old female with a history of inpatient hospitalization for severe depression (including suicide attempts, PTSD due to childhood sexual abuse, and insomnia). Because in the early months of treatment the client's symptoms were overwhelming and talking was too much for her, Visceglia used *pranayama*. As the client's symptoms of depression were intermingled with agitation, Visceglia selected calmer, more grounding breaths, rather than more stimulating breathing exercises.

It was only as the client began feeling safer that Visceglia started adding basic standing poses with awareness of breath and body, guiding the client to stay present with the physical and emotional experiences she encountered. Visceglia guided her client through simple movements such as feeling her feet supporting her body beneath her, inhaling as she moved to stand on tiptoes, and exhaling back to flat feet. Visceglia continued to begin the time together with *pranayama*, a "check-in" of how she felt physically, and simple *asanas*.

This experience points to the crucial role that *pranayama* can have in helping a client to ground. Open-eyed *pranayama* can be helpful for building dual attention with emphasis on both exteroception and interoception. The three most important elements to keep in mind with regard to using *pranayama* for grounding are:

- As mentioned earlier, keep the eyes open at all times. If the client is tempted to close his eyes, invite him to open them, explaining that open eyes lead to a different type of practice.
- Allow both the inhale and the exhale to be through the nose. Inhaling or exhaling through the mouth shifts energy levels and temperature.
- Allow the inhale and exhale to be equally long. Lengthening or abbreviating one vis-à-vis the other shifts energy levels and temperature. Inhaling and exhaling evenly optimizes heart rate variability (HRV) and sympatho-vagal balance (Streeter et al., 2017), and "is both energizing and relaxing, activating first the sympathetic system and then the parasympathetic one, back and forth, in a gentle rhythm" (Mendius & Hanson, 2009, p. 60).

Alternate Nostril Breathing

Alternate nostril breathing is a balancing breath, but do be aware that it can cause anxiety for some people. If you are familiar with this breath, you will see that this variation is a little atypical, as it suggests resting the index and middle fingers on the forehead, for additional grounding. Make sure to remember to invite your client to blow her nose before she starts.

Sit in a position that is comfortable. Place your palms so that they are touching your lap. Keep your eyes open. Inhale for a count of two, reaching the crown of the head towards the ceiling. Exhale for a count of two, relaxing the shoulders. Repeat twice.

Block your right nostril with the thumb of your right hand. Place the index and middle fingers of your right hand in the space between your eyebrows.

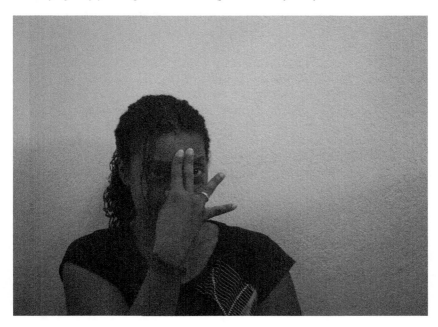

Figure 5.10

Inhale through the left nostril for a count of two, reaching the crown of the head towards the ceiling. Release the thumb from the right nostril, and cover the left nostril with the ring finger of the right hand as you exhale through the right nostril for a count of two, relaxing the shoulders.

Inhale through the right nostril for a count of two, reaching the crown of the head towards the ceiling. Release the ring finger from the left nostril, and cover the right nostril with the thumb as you exhale through the left nostril for a count of two, relaxing the shoulders.

Repeat twice.

Check in with your client, asking, *"What is one word that describes how your body feels right now?"*

Sun Breaths

Sit with your hands by your sides. Inhale and bring the arms to the sides and overhead. Let the palms come together.

Exhale, bringing the palms to the heart center. Repeat twice more.

Tratak

Open-eyed meditation is referred to as "*tratak.*"

Inhale for a count of two, reaching the crown of the head towards the ceiling. Exhale for a count of two, relaxing the shoulders. Repeat for a couple of rounds.

Return to your natural breathing pattern. Notice an object straight ahead of you. Move your eyes to the right, and notice an object there. Now move your eyes to the left, and notice an object there.

Now bring your gaze to a point directly in front of you on the floor. With the next breath, as you breathe in, think of the words, "I am." As you breathe out, think of the word, "present." Continue with this mantra, breathing in and thinking "I am," and breathing out and thinking "present." Continue for a few rounds.

We're going now to release the mantra. Keep your eyes open. Inhale for a count of two, reaching the crown of the head towards the ceiling. Exhale for a count of two, relaxing the shoulders. Repeat four times.

Check in with your client, asking, "*What is one word that describes how your body feels right now?*"

Notice that this practice has several stages to it, to keep your client engaged and present. Make sure his eyes stay open, and that yours do as well. Watch for your client's breath, facial expression, and muscle tightness, as these all provide clues to what is happening. Do not rely on the one word with which they provide you as the sole indication of their experience. Make sure that you keep the breath cycle brief at first, adding repetitions only after you have observed how it affected your client not only during session, but also afterwards.

Grounding for PTSD

Throughout this chapter, we have emphasized the centrality of grounding, both as a starting point and for imbalances that involve mixed *mudha/ksipta* presentations and/or a disconnect from reality. Especially relevant here is PTSD. As we mentioned in Chapter 2, PTSD is a complex psychological injury, in which the brain believes that it is somewhere other than in the here and now. Cortisol is released into the brain, making fight or flight responses easier to "turn on" when a stimulus similar to the traumatic stimulus is present. As a result, the person reexperiences the emotions associated with the trauma, including possible dissociation. Therefore, when working with clients with PTSD, you have to be especially mindful of grounding and emphasizing the here and now, otherwise you can do actual harm.

With this information in mind, there are practices – some of which we have previously discussed as wise to sidestep in general – that are particularly important to avoid when working with clients with symptoms of PTSD:

- Turning off the lights.
- Inviting participants to close their eyes.

- Placing participants in poses where they cannot see the door.
- Placing participants in poses from which it takes longer to come out.
- Telling people how to feel, including in a pose.
- Hands-on assists.
- Poses that encourage vulnerability, such as *savasana* or seated/reclined poses where the legs are in a V-shape.

Poses where the legs are in a V-shape can be triggering for clients who have experienced sexual abuse or assault. You may recall that in Chapter 2 we mentioned that one out of every four girls and one out of every six boys has experienced abuse before the age of 18, and then there are those who experienced assault as adults as well. There are plenty of other poses to practice where the legs are not spread apart in this manner.

Notice that standing poses are helpful here, but in poses where the client turns her head (for example, Warrior II), make sure that you have the client shift positioning so she is facing the door with that turn. Avoid at first poses where it is impossible to watch the door during both the preparation and the hold, such as downward-facing dog – which also takes a little longer to release.

It is helpful to establish a soothing practice for clients with PTSD for times when they feel overwhelmed. Note that this would not be what we might think of as soothing in a general population yoga class – nothing along the lines of closing the eyes and taking a few breaths. Rather, it would be something externally focused, perhaps a round of the 54321 grounding technique to shift awareness into the here and now.

Savasana

If you are a yoga therapist, you may wish to end your practice with your client in *savasana*. Notice that a typical *savasana* does not aim for grounding at all. Therefore, here an open-eyed *savasana* with muscular contraction/ release is far more appropriate. You want it to be balancing, and for a client who is dissociating in any way, a longer *savasana* will be too much. Therefore, this *savasana* should take no longer than three minutes from start to finish. In addition to the more typical option of lying on the back, it includes options of lying on the belly or staying seated, both of which may feel safer, especially for sexual assault and/or abuse survivors. **Do not do *savasana* with someone with symptoms of PTSD.** If you are doing it by yourself, set a timer for three minutes before you begin what follows.

Come either to a position lying on the floor on your back or your belly, or to a comfortable seated position. If you are seated, bring your hands to your lap. If you are lying down, allow your arms to be at your sides. They can be close to your body (which keeps you warmer) or further from your body (which cools you down more). Keep your eyes open, and focus on a point on the ceiling or the floor.

Notice how your body feels here for a second. Then go ahead and contract your feet, as if you're trying to pick something off the floor. Contract tightly, inhale deeply through the nose, and then as you exhale through the mouth, release the contraction.

Now flex your feet, bringing a contraction to the backs of your legs. Tighten all your other leg muscles (contracting your quads, hamstrings, thighs, and calves) as much as you can. Inhale deeply through the nose, and then as you exhale through the mouth, release the contraction.

Contract your buttocks (glutes) very tightly, even lifting them up off the floor if that feels ok for your lower back. Inhale deeply through the nose, and then as you exhale through the mouth, release the contraction.

Notice how your lower body feels, and how your upper body feels.

Contract your abs. Inhale deeply through the nose, and then as you exhale through the mouth, release the contraction.

Make tight fists with your hands, and tighten the muscles in your arms – your biceps and triceps. Inhale deeply through the nose, and then as you exhale through the mouth, release the contraction.

Finally, bring your shoulders towards your ears, and tightly contract your facial muscles, puckering up your eyes, your nose, and the muscles in your jaw area. Inhale deeply through the nose, and then as you exhale through the mouth, release the contraction.

Pause in stillness for a couple of breaths. Let your breath flow smoothly, inhaling and exhaling through the nose.

Begin to bring movement to your fingers and your toes. Make the movement a little larger, rotating your hands and feet. Then make it even larger, moving your entire arm, entire leg, in any way that feels comfortable. Roll over to one side, rest your head on your hand or arm if you like. Then place your other palm on the floor, and press into it to bring yourself up to a comfortable seated position.

Check in with your client, asking, "*What is one word that describes how your body feels right now?*"

Closing the Practice

In contrast with a typical yoga class, even if you choose to do a *savasana* of this nature, it should not be where you end your grounding practice. Instead, now you want to orient the client back to the surrounding space. She will leave your office and most likely get in the car and drive, and you want her to be present in the here and now. The 54321 grounding technique is an excellent way to do that.

If you are a psychotherapist, this will be a sufficient set of practices for you and your client in session, as you presumably will engage in other therapy modalities also. While you may want to begin with the orientation practices at the start of the session, there are varying advantages to including the *asanas* and *pranayamas* towards the start or towards the end. At the start they set a more grounded tone, but the client risks losing that benefit as she begins talking about the story and returning to more familiar lines. Towards the end allows the client to leave the session feeling more grounded, but you and the client may have to set up a clear framework for when you will begin the yoga portion of your session so that it does not feel abrupt or rushed. Either way, it is definitely helpful to end with one *asana* and one *pranayama*, so that the client feels grounded before leaving.

If you are a yoga therapist, this chapter will provide guidance for you on what else you might like to introduce in your session. Moving gradually will mean that you might have more time at the start, so perhaps after the session in which you do intake, you can schedule shorter sessions for a while as you build up. Resist the temptation to pack more in if the client seems to be feeling grounded; you need to observe how things unfold from session to session. Practice shifting away from the cues that you typically use to assess "progress" (an aligned outward form) and language/physical assists that are aimed towards extending further physically in the pose, and instead, continuously check in with your goal here: building grounding. In what way does each practice you introduce contribute to that? Notice if your inclination is to bring in poses that are more challenging for the sake of physical mastery, and if you are losing sight of your emotional health focus by doing that.

With that in mind, think of what other practices you may wish to introduce over time. What would serve to ground the client further, if further grounding is appropriate? Keep in mind the contact with the floor, the straight lines of the body, and maintaining symmetry. Notice how much hip opening is required for each pose that you consider, and how hip opening is generally at odds with grounding. Notice how much balance is required for the pose, and how balance is generally at odds with grounding.

As we mentioned earlier, you will continue with a grounding practice for your dissociative and mixed symptom clients. But for your other clients, once you have observed that they maintain grounding through the variety of practices presented in this chapter, it may now be time to see if they are ready to proceed to a *brahmana* or *langhana* practice.

Vignette

Sarah, a 27-year-old female, came to see me because of a variety of issues in her marriage, with her parents, and at her work. She was energetic and engaging, and the front desk staff at the place where I was working at the time loved her. However, beneath that exterior she could turn to anger and blame quickly. I discovered this one day when the receptionist had to attend to something else, and so took a little longer to check her in. Sarah, who in the past had had high praise for the receptionist, was now furious, shouting and cursing at and about her as she came in to my office for her session.

At the time, I was still beginning to experiment with working with yoga directly for emotional health imbalance, and so I suggested to Sarah that she close her eyes and take long, deep breaths. She closed her eyes for a mini-second, and then immediately they flew open again. "That b_____! Why would she do that? This has been such a s_____ week. My boss told me that I was rude to this one customer. She's the one who's rude. She_____."

From here began a tirade against her boss. While at the time I had not yet developed the Three-Pronged Model to inform me right away, I saw that Sarah was not in an emotionally stable place. So as she was talking, I said in a calm voice, "Let's go ahead and stand up," and did so myself, standing with my feet hip-width apart and arms by my side. She stood up, emulating my stance as she continued talking. But as she came into position, her talking began to slow down.

Without a word, I brought my arms up to shoulder level, and then all the way up to Mountain pose. Sarah did the same, now talking much more slowly.

"You can keep telling me what happened," I said, "while at the same time letting your gaze focus on a point in front of you on the floor. As you breathe in, reach your fingertips up towards the ceiling. As you breathe out, relax your shoulders."

Sarah paused mid-story to synchronize her breath and movements with my instructions. And as she did that, she exhaled, and then came into silence.

"Take three more breaths here. And now, take five breaths to bring your arms down by your sides," I said, following her pace and moving my arms down slowly as well. "Keep your gaze on the point in front of you. What's one word that describes how your body feels right now?"

"Calm," Sarah said.

As you're reading about Sarah, some of you may recognize several signs of borderline personality disorder: the intense emotionality, external blaming, and swinging between emotional extremes. But even if you do not recognize those symptoms, you can see that when Sarah came in she was not only highly agitated, but also ungrounded. Her emotions were intense and unstable. When I tried to guide her to close her eyes, she was unable to do so.

Notice that meeting Sarah where she was meant connecting with her in that verbally agitated state. If I had tried to stop the flow of her words, chances are I would have ended up being at the receiving end of her anger. Rather, I held space for her words while gently guiding our movements: *"You can keep telling me what happened, while at the same time letting your gaze focus on a point in front of you on the floor."* I then gave her a movement/breath pattern to which to attend: *"As you breathe in, reach your fingertips up towards the ceiling. As you breathe out, relax your shoulders."* In effect, I was asking Sarah to pat her head and rub her belly at the same time: as she shifted away from sympathetic nervous system agitation and into parasympathetic nervous system stimulation, it became increasingly difficult for her to main her aroused state.

Notice that I was also able to guide Sarah here because of the relationship that the two of us had established. If we had not had a relationship, chances are she would not have been willing to be guided while in such an agitated and distracted state. That is the factor that cannot be measured in research evidence, but is ultimately what makes or breaks the therapeutic experience.

References

da Silva, T. L., Ravindran, L. N., & Ravindran, A. V. (2009). Yoga in the treatment of mood and anxiety disorders: A review. *Asian Journal of Psychiatry, 2*(1), 6–16. doi: 10.1016/j.ajp.2008.12.002

Mendius, R., & Hanson, R. (2009) *Buddha's brain: The practical neuroscience of happiness, love & wisdom*. Oakland, CA: New Harbinger Publications.

Streeter, C. C., Gerbarg, P. L., Whitfield, T. H., Owen, L., Johnston, J., Silveri, M. M., … Jensen, J. E. (2017). Treatment of major depressive disorder with Iyengar yoga and coherent breathing: A randomized controlled dosing study. *Journal of Alternative and Complementary Medicine, 23*(3), 201–207. doi: 10.1089/acm.2016.0140

Uebelacker, L., Weinstock, L., & Kraines, M. (2014). Self-reported benefits and risks of yoga in individuals with bipolar disorder. *Journal of Psychiatric Practice, 20*(5), 345–352. doi: 10.1097/01.pra.0000454779.59859.f8

van der Kolk, B. A. (2015). *The body keeps the score: Brain, mind, and body in the healing of trauma*. New York, NY: Penguin Books.

Visceglia, E. (2015). Psychiatry and yoga therapy. In L. Payne, T. Gold, E. Goldman, & C. Rosenberg (Eds.), *Yoga therapy & integrative medicine: Where ancient science meets modern medicine* (pp. 143–155). Laguna Beach, CA: Basic Health Publications.

6   Building Energy and Vitality

If we are working with a client who is experiencing a dulling of energy (*mudha*), then after we are receiving consistent feedback that indicates stability in the grounding practices from Chapter 5, we may move to weaving in some *brahmana* practices that build energy. In the words of one yoga teacher: "A good yoga practice … involved poses that cycled through the accelerator and the brake so that the autonomic system got a thorough workout" (Broad, 2012, p. 95). During a *brahmana* practice, we are working the accelerator. But if we press it too hard, the car will spin out of control and possibly crash. Just like pushing the pedal to the metal wears a car out, accelerating too fast will do the same for your client.

Who Benefits from a *Brahmana* Practice?

As a *brahmana* practice addresses *mudha*, it is optimal for imbalances, such as major depressive disorder and persistent depressive disorder, that come with melancholic features. As we mentioned in the previous chapters, it is not appropriate when depression exists alongside a *ksipta*-related condition such as anxiety, or the potential mania/hypomania present in bipolar disorders.

What Does a *Brahmana* Practice Entail?

A *brahmana* practice involves building energy, which typically correlates with creating heat. It includes the following:

- Breaths where the inhale is longer than the exhale, including those that involve a regular inhale through the nose and a rapid exhale through the mouth.
- Combining holding a grounding pose with a faster breath pattern.
- Poses that involve a backbend.
- Visualizations of building energy and inviting in desired qualities.
- Having the eyes open, to focus on the here and now. Closing the eyes during *mudha* can lead to a retreat into a dark inner world with many

stories, whereas keeping them open helps the client to remain in the present while working to build energy and vitality.

- A morning practice, in order to set the tone for the day. However, it can be beneficial to return to it later in the day on an as-needed basis, but not five hours or less before bedtime, as it might raise energy at a time when a person should be winding down. If you are guiding a client experiencing *mudha*, keep this in mind when scheduling sessions.

Of course, we can also encourage *brahmana* via a more vigorous flow, or a faster breath such as *bhastrika* or *kapalabhati*/breath of fire. But then we are risking pressing the accelerator too hard and burning the client out.

Beginning the Practice: *Asanas*

As you shift to *brahmana*, always start your session with grounding poses and breaths. If, about ten minutes into your grounding practices, your client responds to "What is one word that describes how you feel in your body?" with answers that consistently indicate stability, you can start introducing *brahmana*. As we did with grounding, we will introduce *brahmana* practices gradually. That means not only that we will initiate no more than a couple of new practices at any one time, but also that we will wait between one session and the next to assess long-term impact on the client before increasing hold time or adding repetitions of the same practice. We will also make sure to end the session with at least five minutes of grounding practice.

In Chapter 4, we mentioned that one of the most important things to keep in mind is where we meet the client. That is especially relevant when we begin to work with *brahmana* and *langhana* practices. If I am working with a client with depression, I know that what we are aiming towards is a build-up of *brahmana*. But if I start at a place of energy that is too high, my client will not be ready to join me there. I remember when I was taking my yoga teacher training, our first practice of the day was at 6 am. Our instructors, who knew that most of us had rolled out of bed 10 minutes beforehand, would typically start on the floor with very slow movements, before very gradually moving us up to standing. They knew that if they started in a place of higher energy, it would feel jarring to us. We want to meet the client where he is, and then start just a tiny step above his energy level.

Warm-Ups

Each of these warm-ups can be tried out independently first to test for the client's window of affect tolerance, before progressing to use them in combination and then as warm-ups before other practices.

Six Movements of the Spine

This sequence allows the client to move the body between three types of paired movements that all start from a position on all fours with a neutral spine. Introduce the first pair of movements (Cat/Cow) to the client and assess the effects of that, then add the second pair (Side Right/Side Left), and then the third pair (Threading the Needle).

CAT/COW

Come to your hands and knees.
    Inhale, pressing into your fingertips. On an exhale, curve your spine into a cat stretch. See Figure 5.4.
    Inhale, coming into Cow pose. See Figure 5.5.
    Exhale, coming into Cat. Repeat each pose twice more.

SIDE RIGHT/SIDE LEFT

Inhale to a flat back. Press into the finger tips. Exhale and look over your right shoulder.
    Inhale back to center. Exhale and look over your left shoulder.
    Repeat twice more on each side.

THREADING THE NEEDLE

Inhale to a flat back, and lift the right arm off the floor, so that the fingertips are facing the ceiling.
    Exhale, sliding the right arm to the floor so that the arm is perpendicular to your spine and the right forearm/right hand comes palm up underneath the left shoulder. Bring the right shoulder and right cheek to touch the floor.
    Inhale the right arm back up. Exhale the right hand back down to the floor.
    Inhale the left arm off the floor, so that the fingertips are facing the ceiling. Exhale, sliding the left arm to the floor so that the arm is perpendicular to your spine and the left forearm/left hand comes palm up underneath the right shoulder. Bring the left shoulder and left cheek to touch the floor.
    Inhale the left arm back up. Exhale the left hand down to the floor.
    Repeat twice more on each side. Come to sit on your heels, and take a breath.
    Check in with your client, asking, "*What is one word that describes how your body feels right now?*"

Notice the types of movements involved in the three parts of this sequence. In the first, the alternation of Cow–Cat tests your client's tolerance of a slight backbend (Cow), which is now practiced right after a slight forward bend (Cat). Repeating this combination three times – as opposed to the one time between grounding poses as we did in the universal warm-up in Chapter 5 – tests things a little more. If that works for your client, then you will explore what it is like for him to combine those movements with moving the spine side-to-side, and then twisting it in Threading the Needle.

Now that we have moved on from grounding, the type of response for which you are looking is different. Rather than a consistent sense of stability, you are listening out for words that indicate an energetic shift, while at the same time pointing to the shift being contained. So your client may say he feels "stable," but he may also say he feels "energized" or "tired." Notice that if he says he feels "tired," then you may have been progressing too fast, and you need to slow down.

If your client says he feels "energized," you want to get a sense of how contained that energy is, as we do not want to unleash energy that is chaotic and in any way overwhelming. Prompt him, "Tell me more about how 'energized' feels." If your client says something that indicates instability ("intense," "ungrounded," "weird," and "distressed" are all responses I have received here), guide him to take a deep breath in and out, and return to grounding without commentary (Do not say, "Since it sounds like your energy is chaotic, we are going to go back to grounding.") Again, remember that the energy may not emerge until after the session, and this is why it is important to proceed gradually, and check in at the next session.

Once your client who has been experiencing *mudha* has tasted some energy, that sample is all he needs at first – no need to provide more. Remember, you are not ramming the accelerator and spinning the car out of control – rather, you are increasing the speed gradually.

After you have combined the movements a pair at a time and know that your client is experiencing relatively contained energy (or is feeling stable and grounded), you can gradually add repetitions of the entire sequence, and see how it affects her. And once she reports feeling contained energy throughout, you may move on to some of the other practices that follow.

Pulling Prana

Pulling *prana* is an excellent way of combining breath with a little movement. You can start with one breath, and check in, and then add a couple more each session, up to a total of six. I am providing three variations of arm movements here, so once you are doing six repetitions with one arm variation and the client reports feeling contained energy, you can move on to adding another variation.

VARIATION 1

Stand with your feet hip-width apart, or if that doesn't work for your body, come into a comfortable, grounded seat.

Reach your arms up so that they are parallel to your ears, as you would in Mountain (see Figure 0.3), while inhaling quickly through the nose.

Exhale through the mouth quickly with a "ha" sound, as you pull the arms down. Repeat twice more.

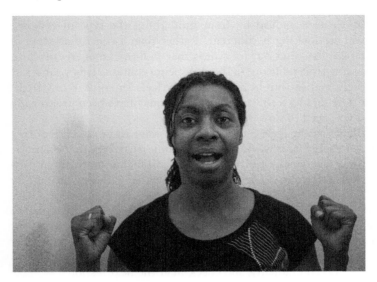

Figure 6.1

Check in with your client, asking, *"What is one word that describes how your body feels right now?"*

VARIATION 2

Stand with your feet hip-width apart, or if that doesn't work for your body, come into a comfortable, grounded seat.

Reach your arms forward, while inhaling quickly through the nose. The arm position is similar to that in Figure 0.1.

Exhale through the mouth quickly with a "ha" sound, as you pull the arms back, bending at the elbows. Repeat twice more.

Check in with your client, asking, *"What is one word that describes how your body feels right now?"*

VARIATION 3

Stand with your feet hip-width apart, or if that doesn't work for your body, come into a comfortable, grounded seat.

Reach your arms to a T-position, palms down, while inhaling quickly through the nose. The arm position is similar to that in Figure 0.2.

Exhale through the mouth quickly with a "ha" sound, as you pull the arms in. Repeat twice more.

Check in with your client, asking, *"What is one word that describes how your body feels right now?"*

Hip Swings

Sit on the floor with your feet in front of you. The soles of the feet are on the floor, and the knees are bent. Your palms are on the floor beside you or behind you.

Inhale, and as you exhale, bring the knees to the right.

Inhale back to center, and exhale bringing your knees to the left. Repeat two more times.

Check in with your client, asking, *"What is one word that describes how your body feels right now?"*

If the client's energy is contained here, you may now guide him through the same movement, but exhaling through the mouth, with a "ha" sound.

Pushing into the Wall

Stand facing the wall. Take a few steps back, and place your hands on the wall. Spread your fingers wide.

Step your right foot forward, and inch your left foot back. Bring the heel of your left foot towards the floor as much as possible. Bend your right knee, and make sure the knee doesn't go past the ankle. Press into your hands. Hold for three breaths. As you inhale, press into your fingers. As you exhale, relax your shoulders. Repeat.

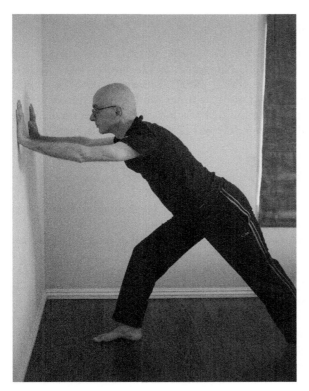

Figure 6.2

Switch feet, and repeat for three breaths.

Check in with your client, asking, *"What is one word that describes how your body feels right now?"*

Once your client has practiced this variation several times and you know that his energy is contained here, you can add a "ha" breath on the exhale.

Step your right foot forward, and inch your left foot back. Bend your right knee, and make sure the knee doesn't go past the ankle. Inhale here. Exhale with a "ha" sound, pressing into your hands. Inhale, releasing the pressure in your hands but keeping them on the wall. Exhale with a "ha" and press into them. Repeat twice.

Check in with your client, asking, *"What is one word that describes how your body feels right now?"*

Beginning and Building the Practice: *Pranayama* and Meditation

There are changes that we can make to the length and type of breath to build energy.

Right Nostril Breathing

Inhaling and exhaling out of the right nostril is warming and energizing to the body (Telles, Nagathna, & Nagendra, 1996; Telles, Raghuraj, Maharana, & Nagendra, 2007). However, do not repeat right nostril breathing more than five times, and always start and end with a few regular breaths through both nostrils, as prompted in the following and as we did in the previous chapter before alternate nostril breathing.

Sit in a position that is comfortable. Place your palms so that they are touching your lap. Keep your eyes open.

Inhale for a count of two, reaching the crown of the head towards the ceiling. Exhale for a count of two, relaxing the shoulders. Repeat twice.

Block your left nostril with the thumb of your left hand. Keep the right hand where it is.

Inhale through the right nostril for a count of two, reaching the crown of the head towards the ceiling. Exhale through the right nostril for a count of two, relaxing the shoulders. Repeat twice.

Release your left hand back to your lap. Notice a word that describes how you feel in your body right now, and keep it in mind without speaking it out loud. Now inhale for a count of two through both nostrils, reaching the crown of the head towards the ceiling. Exhale for a count of two through both nostrils, relaxing the shoulders. Repeat twice.

Check in with your client, asking, "*What is one word that describes how your body feels right now? And what was the word that described how you felt right after breathing through the right nostril?*"

This is the first time that we have asked the client to think of a word and retain it. There are very few times when we do this, as we do not want the client to be so concerned about remembering words that she stops being in the moment.

Inhale with Visualization

Another way to energize the body is by increasing the length of the inhale relative to the length of the exhale. This is a practice that can be effective for the seasoned practitioner, but potentially overwhelming and anxiety provoking for the novice. Therefore, instead of focusing on the length of the inhale, we can emphasize it by adding a visualization.

Come into a comfortable seated position, with both hands on your lap.

Think of a quality that you would like to feel more in your life (e.g., love, joy, or light). Check in with your client, "*What might that feeling be?*" *Now, as you breathe in through the nose, imagine yourself filling with* _____ (insert the feeling here). *As you breathe out through the nose, notice your body. Again, breathe in, imagine yourself filling with* _____. *As you breathe out through the nose, notice your body. Now continue three more times at your own pace.*

Check in with your client, asking, "*What is one word that describes how your body feels right now?*"

Here you want to make sure that the feeling that your client names is in the affirmative, not in the negative. So if she says she does not want to be anxious anymore, specifically ask her how she would like to feel instead (e.g., calm or happy) and use that word.

Bhramari *(Bee Breath) with* Padma Mudra

This breath can be energizing or calming, depending on the person practicing, and we will therefore encounter it again in the next chapter on *langhana*. There, we will use the traditional hand variation, whereas here, we will adopt an alternative on which the client can focus his gaze. This helps him to be more in the present rather than drawing inwards. You can look up *bhramari* on YouTube to get a sense of how it might sound.

Bring the palms together in front of the heart center.

Keep the thumbs and pinky fingers together, but separate the other fingers. This is padma mudra. Look at your hands, and inhale. On an exhale, begin humming. When you run out of breath, inhale and start again.

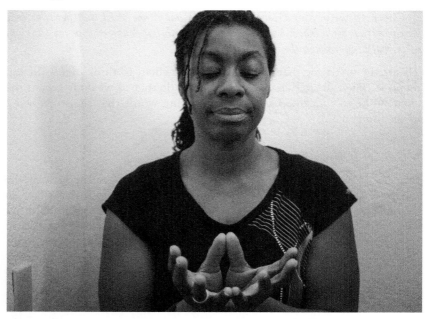

Figure 6.3

Check in with your client, asking, *"What is one word that describes how your body feels right now?"*

As the effects of this breath may differ, if you find that it is calming for your client, then you know that this is not part of a *brahmana* practice for him.

Breath of Joy

We encountered the breath of joy in the introduction, and now it is time to revisit it. See the Introduction for photos of the different arm variations.

Raise your arms so they're at shoulder level, directly in front of you, while inhaling quickly through the nose.

Raise your arms so they're at shoulder level, out in a T-position, while inhaling a second time quickly through the nose.

Raise your arms so they're overhead, while inhaling a third time quickly through the nose.

Exhale forcefully through the mouth with a "ha" and bend all the way forward, so that the crown of your head is reaching down towards the floor. If you are sitting in a chair, bend your torso forward so that it hangs between your feet. If you have unmedicated high or low blood pressure or you are pregnant, make sure that your breaths are not as forceful, and also only bend forward till your torso is parallel with the floor (i.e., at no more than 90 degrees from your legs if you're standing).

Come back up, and repeat this breath four more times in a row. Allow your arms to swing from one arm position to the next.

Check in with your client, asking, *"What is one word that describes how your body feels right now?"*

As your client becomes more familiar with this breath, you may guide her to move through it faster if that is comfortable for her body.

Tratak

In line with our open-eyed focus for a *brahmana* practice, the meditation we practice will still be *tratak*. Gazing at a candle (whether real or artificial) can be helpful here, as the flame of a real candle in particular evokes warmth and energy.

Keeping your eyes open, allow your gaze to fall softly on the wick of a candle. Keep your gaze there, as you take ten breaths through the nose.

You can guide your client to add time up to 20 breaths as time goes on.

Building the Practice: *Asanas*

Standing Poses Category 2 – Poses Emphasizing Heat

In Chapter 5, we discussed a series of standing poses that included a solid base along with a more energizing side-to-side movement, a slight backbend in the torso, and/or a deeper opening in the hips. These include Half Moon (*Ardha Chandrasana*), Goddess (*Utkata Konasana*), Triangle (*Trikonasana*), Crescent (*Anjaneyasana*), Warrior I (*Virabhadrasana* I), Reverse Warrior (*Viparita Virabhadrasana*), Revolved Triangle (*Parivrtta Trikonasana*), and Revolved Side Angle (*Parivrtta Parsvakonasana*). We will encounter the first four of these in the moon salutations that follow.

Moon Salutations

Some styles of yoga do not practice at the time of a full moon, others shift the practice somewhat, and still others incorporate specific sequences referred to as moon salutations. This version of moon salutations is from the Kripalu tradition, except that I have omitted one pose (*malasana*/Garland pose), which puts pressure on the knees and therefore may cause injury in someone whose body has not been trained appropriately.

Moon salutations can be energizing for a client experiencing *mudha*, but in a cooler manner than the more heat-inducing sun salutations. The sequence is composed of performing a set of poses on the right side of the body, and then performing them in reverse order on the left side of the body. This sequencing mirrors the phases of the moon, waxing till the full moon and then waning back till the dark preceding the new moon.

Make sure to introduce the poses to your client gradually, practicing a couple of them at a time on each side and seeing how they impact her.

Coming to the center of your space, stand with your feet hip-width apart.

Inhale, bringing the arms up by the ears.

Half Moon, right: *Exhale, interlacing the fingers together with the forefingers touching (steeple position). Press out through the left hip, coming down to the right. Note that the movement comes from the hip, rather than from scrunching the spine. If having the arms in this position doesn't work for you, you can bring one arm or both arms on your hip or by your side. In any of the variations, make sure that the shoulders are relaxed.*

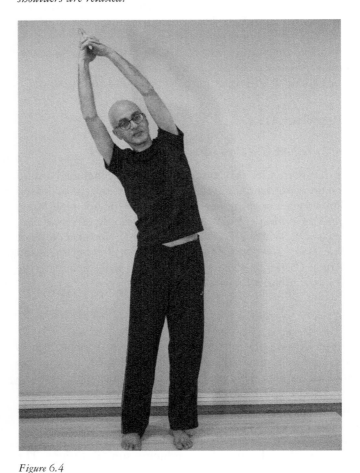

Figure 6.4

Inhale, coming back to center, with the arms staying as they are.

Half Moon, left: *Exhale and press out through the right hip, coming down to the left. Again, note that the movement comes from the hip, rather than from scrunching the spine. And again, if having the arms in this position doesn't work for you, you can bring one arm or both arms on your hip or by your side. Make sure that the shoulders are relaxed.*

Inhale, coming back to center.

Exhale, stepping one foot out wide, to the five-pointed star. The arms are at shoulder level, palms down.

Goddess: *Turn the feet out as much towards 90 degrees as works for you. Bend into the knees as deeply as works for you, and widen the distance between your feet so that the knees don't go past the toes. Bend at the elbows. The palms can face each other, or face forward, coming into Goddess pose.*

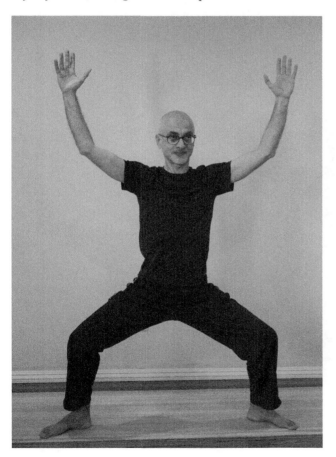

Figure 6.5

Turn your right foot out 90 degrees, and your left foot in 15–30 degrees. Press out through the left hip, and reach out through the fingers of the right hand.

Triangle: *Windmill your arms, so that the back of the right hand rests on the right leg, and the fingertips of the left hand reach up towards the ceiling. You can also have a block behind the right foot, and place your right hand there. If it doesn't work to have the left arm up, you can have the left hand on the left hip. You can look up at the left hand or down at the right foot, or if that doesn't work for your neck, then look straight ahead.*

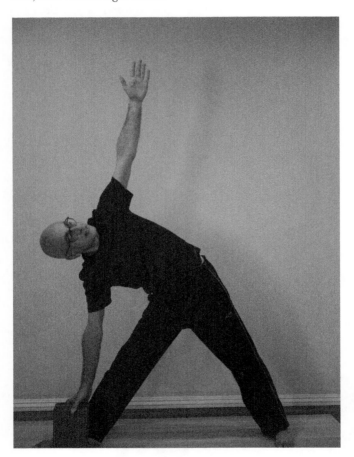

Figure 6.6

Pyramid: *Turn your body to face your right leg. Make sure there is a slight bend in it, then bring your hands onto the floor on either side of your right foot, on blocks on either side of your right foot, or on your right leg (anywhere but on the knee). If you have high or low blood pressure, keep the head and neck in line with the heart; otherwise, bring the forehead towards the leg, coming into pyramid pose.*

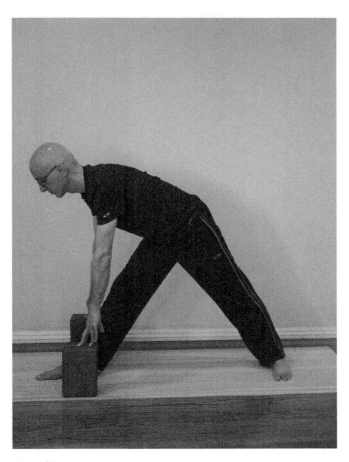

Figure 6.7

Lunge: *Bend into the right knee, and come to the toes of the left foot. Widen the distance between your feet if necessary so that the right knee is in a straight line with the right ankle. Keep the hands on either side of the right foot, on the floor or on blocks, coming into a high lunge.*

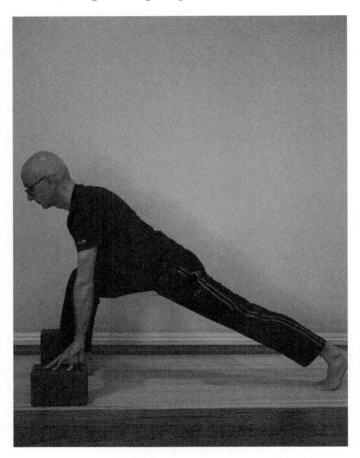

Figure 6.8

Bring the right hand between the right foot and the left hand. If you were using blocks, take them with you.

Turn your body to face forward, and walk the hands towards the center. If you were using blocks, keep taking them with you.

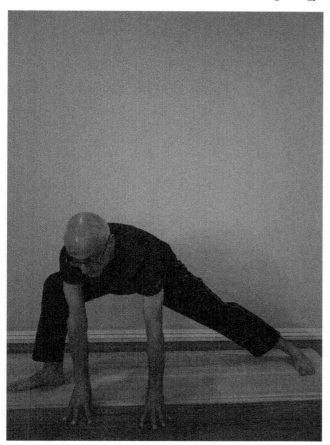

Figure 6.9

    You will now come into the same movements, but in reverse order, on the left side.
Lunge: *Walk the hands over to the other side, and come into the high lunge on the left side. The hands are now on either side of the left foot, on the floor or on blocks.*
Pyramid: *Bring the heel of the right foot on the floor, so that the right foot is turned in 15–30 degrees. The left foot is still out 90 degrees. Your hands are on the floor on either side of your left foot, on blocks on either side of your left foot, or on your left leg (anywhere but on the knee). If you have high or low blood pressure, keep the head and neck in line with the heart; otherwise, bring the forehead towards the leg, coming into pyramid pose.*

Triangle: *Bring the left hand on the left leg, and reach the right arm up towards the ceiling, coming into triangle. You can also place your left hand on a block behind your left foot. If it doesn't work to have the right arm up, you can have the right hand on the left hip. You can look up at the right hand or down at the left foot, or if that doesn't work for your neck, then look straight ahead.*

Goddess: *Bring your torso up, and turn the right foot out as much towards 90 degrees as works for you. Bend into the knees as deeply as works for you, and widen the distance between your feet so that the knees don't go past the toes. Bend at the elbows. The palms can face each other, or face forward, coming into Goddess pose.*

Straighten your legs, and turn your feet to face forward. Straighten your arms so that they are at shoulder level, palms down.

Step the feet hip-width apart from each other. Bring the arms up by your ears.

Half Moon, left: *Exhale, interlacing the fingers together with the forefingers touching (steeple position). Press out through the right hip coming down to the left. If having the arms in this position doesn't work for you, you can bring one arm or both arms on your hip or by your side. Make sure that the shoulders are relaxed.*

Inhale, coming back to center, with the arms staying as they are.

Half Moon, right: *Exhale and press out through the left hip, coming down to the right. If having the arms in this position doesn't work for you, you can bring one arm or both arms on your hip or by your side. Make sure that the shoulders are relaxed.*

Inhale, coming back to center.

Exhale, release the hands down by your sides, then bring the palms together in front of the heart center.

Check in with your client, asking, "*What is one word that describes how your body feels right now?*"

After you have gone through the individual postures separately with your client and found out the following week how that impacted him, you can move on to the entire sequence. And when you have feedback about that, you can increase repetitions of the entire sequence, one round at a time.

Once your client is up to five repetitions, you may wish to add other poses at the lunge juncture, if your client is interested in a more physically intense practice. Note that in order for a practice to be more challenging, that does not mean that you need to introduce what we tend to think of as more "advanced" poses. Rather, we will come from the lunge to crescent pose, and add variations here.

From the high lunge (Figure 6.8):

Keeping the legs as they are, bring your hands onto your right quad, and raise the torso up to vertical.

Bring the arms up by your ears. This is Crescent pose.

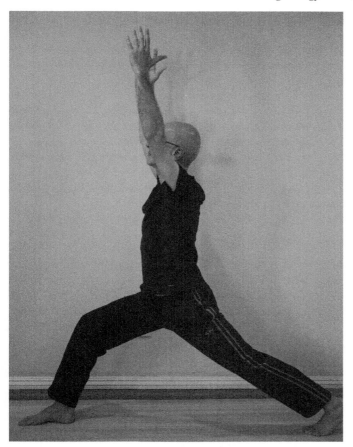

Figure 6.10

From here, we will work to energize the body by staying in the lunge position, but experimenting with different arm variations. These arm variations can be tried one at a time.

Add-on 1: *Bring the hands in front of the heart.*
Add-on 2: *Bring the arms to a T-position.*
Add-on 3: *Clasp alternate elbows.*
Add-on 4: *Bring the palms together in front of the heart center. Twist to your right, placing the left elbow outside the right leg. Press the left arm into the right leg, to gain more range and leverage in the twist.*

If the energy continues to be contained for your client as she practices these arm variations, then you may combine them into sequences such as the one following. If your client wishes, he can also involve the back leg in the combination, bringing a slight bend into the knee on the exhale, and inhaling it to straight again.

Add-on combination 1: *Inhale, bring the arms by your ears. Exhale, bring the arms to a T-position. Inhale, bring the arms up by your ears. Exhale, clasp alternate elbows. Repeat up to three times.*

Add-on combination 2: *Inhale, bring the arms by your ears. Exhale, bring the arms to a T-position. Inhale, bring the arms up by your ears. Exhale, clasp alternate elbows. Inhale, bring the arms in front of the heart center. Exhale, twist to your right, place the left elbow outside the right leg. Repeat up to three times.*

Return to the lunge, bringing the hands down to the floor, and proceed through the moon salutation. Repeat the add-on(s) after the lunge on the left side.

Remember that your aim is not to tire your client, but to energize him, so as usual, add gradually and check in frequently.

Synchronizing Breath with Movement

You can combine an energizing breath such as that of pulling *prana* (inhale through the nose, exhale with a "ha" through the mouth) with any grounding pose for more energy. Just make sure that there is some sort of arm movement on the exhale.

Warrior II with Pulling Prana Arms

One example of that is to guide the client into Warrior II, then add the following:

With your arms at shoulder level, palms down, inhale and reach through the fingertips.

Exhale with a "ha" through the mouth, pulling the arms close to the body, as we did on the exhale for pulling prana. *Repeat twice more.*

Check in with your client, asking, *"What is one word that describes how your body feels right now?"*

Backbends (not Forward Bends)

In many ways, backbends are the "gold standard" in yoga when it comes to addressing depression. However, as I have repeatedly emphasized, it is important to build up to doing them. We have encountered Cow pose – a slight backbend – in both the universal warm-up and the six positions of the spine. As you have arrived at this portion of the practice, it means that your client was able to be grounded while moving through them.

Since we never want to lose our grounding even when working to energize, our backbends all start from a position on the floor, and the body maintains a strong degree of contact with the floor throughout. Also significantly, the neck is only at a slight curve from the top of the spine, further maintaining the grounding effect. As with everything, we will build up slowly, exploring the effects of both an active and a passive backbend. In an active backbend, the client is using his own body strength to hold the backbend. In a passive backbend, she is being supported by something else, such as props. Active backbends generally allow more energetic build-up, whereas passive ones allow release.

Active Backbend: Sphynx

Come to a position lying down on the belly, with your palms on either side of your chest.

Press into your lower body, and on an exhale, lift your hands and torso off the floor. Notice how this affects your back.

If the lift didn't feel right for your back, then lower down slowly. Backbends of this nature are not the right thing for your body right now. If lifting felt fine for your back, then bring your forearms onto the floor, with the elbows directly below the shoulders, coming into Sphynx pose. Hold here for three breaths. As you inhale, press the forearms (not the elbows) into the floor. As you exhale, relax the shoulders.

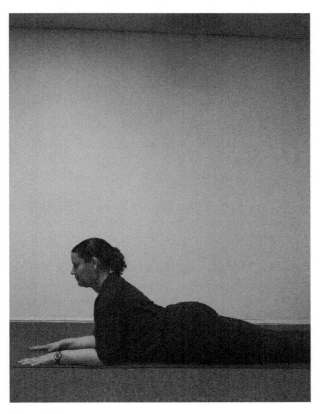

Figure 6.11

Lift the elbows off the floor, and slowly lower the torso to the floor.

Turn your head to one side. Bend your knees, windshield wiping your legs from side to side as a countermovement for the lower back.

Check in with your client, asking, "*What is one word that describes how your body feels right now?*" The emphasis on pressing the forearms into the floor on the inhale and relaxing the shoulders on the exhale keeps the client present in the moment and engaged. You never want your client who has been experiencing emotional distress just to "hang out" in a pose, and especially not a backbend. For a yoga therapist or a psychotherapist who has been practicing yoga for a long time, holding a pose within an expanse of silence can feel therapeutic, but that may not be the case when one's inner world is a challenging one. It is better to err on the side of not allowing enough silence at the start than to allow too much and lose the client from the present moment.

Check in with your client the following week to assess the longer-term effects of Sphynx on her body and emotions. If the pose was emotionally and physically viable, you may wish to explore Cobra. Highlight that Sphynx, as a backbend, also moves energy, and so staying with it is still emotionally effective. Remember and remind your client that this is not a typical yoga experience where your focus is to build back strength; rather, the aim is to shift *mudha* and build vitality in as safe a way as possible.

Active Backbend: Cobra

Come to a position lying down on the floor, with your palms on either side of your chest.

Press into your lower body, and on an exhale, lift your hands and torso off the floor. Notice how this affects your back.

If the lift didn't feel right for your back, then lower down slowly. Backbends of this nature are not the right thing for your body right now. If lifting felt fine for your back, then bring your hands back down onto the floor on either side of your chest, with the fingers spread wide. Move your shoulders away from your ears. Continue pressing into your fingers, lifting your torso up, as long as you don't feel pressure in your lower back. If at any point you do, very slowly come back down. Hold your expression of Cobra for three breaths, looking straight ahead (not tilting the head back). As you inhale, press the fingers (not the wrists) into the floor. As you exhale, relax the shoulders.

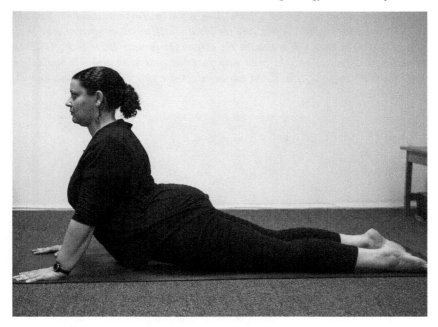

Figure 6.12

To release, very slowly lower down. Turn your head to one side. Bend your knees, windshield wiping your legs from side to side as a countermovement for the lower back.

Check in with your client, asking, *"What is one word that describes how your body feels right now?"*

Note that in this hold of Cobra, we are guiding the client not to tilt the head back, in order to further maintain grounding.

Active Backbend: Bridge

If/once your client has contained energy in Sphynx and/or Cobra, you may try Bridge, a more vulnerable pose as the hips and pelvis are exposed.

Come to lie on your back, with your knees bent and your feet on the floor. Make sure that your feet are hip-width apart, that is, the front of your hip is in line with the midpoint of your knee. Bring your arms by your sides, and make sure you can touch your heels with your fingertips. Place a block between your inner thighs.

Bring your arms back by your sides. Press into your feet, and lift your tailbone off the floor. Notice how that feels in your back. If it feels ok, raise the rest of your lower back off the floor. If that feels ok, raise your midback, then your upper back. If at any point something doesn't feel right in your back, lower down to the version that felt fine.

If having your upper back off the floor is ok, walk your shoulders in, and clasp your hands together. Make sure the block is still in place between your inner thighs – it is helping you maintain the alignment in your lower body. Hold for three breaths. As you inhale, press into your feet and your arms. If you'd like, press the block in place as well. As you exhale, raise your belly button towards the ceiling. Repeat.

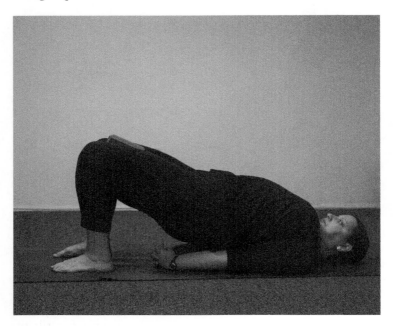

Figure 6.13

If you clasped your hands, unclasp them, and bring your arms by your sides. Press into your arms, and slowly release your spine down to the floor, one vertebra at a time, from the upper to the lower spine. When your spine is all the way on the floor, bring your knees into your chest, and rock your hips side to side.

Check in with your client, asking, *"What is one word that describes how your body feels right now?"*

Be particularly attentive as you guide your client in this pose. Amy Weintraub describes a release of tears that occurred for her in this pose: "these were not tears of pain, nor were they triggered by conscious memory. My body was simply letting go of something it had held on to for far too long" (2004, p. 215). She emphasizes how the pose taps into emotional vulnerability; "because the pelvis and chest areas are lifted and unprotected, this pose can bring up repressed emotion – fear is not uncommon, particularly in someone who may have been sexually traumatized" (p. 214)

Passive Backbend: Supported Fish

Take a yoga blanket, and roll it up tightly along the long edge.

Place the rolled blanket towards the back of your yoga mat. It should be placed lengthways, so that it is parallel to the long edge of the mat, with the fringed edge facing the back of the mat. Sit in front of it, with about a hand's length away from its edge.

Lie down on the blanket so that it is directly underneath your spine. If you like, fold the top of it underneath your head as a pillow. Hold for five breaths. As you inhale, notice the contact between your back and the blanket. As you exhale, relax the body. Repeat.

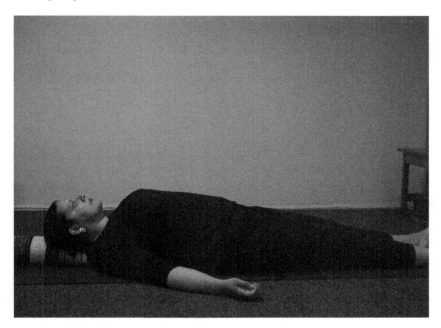

Figure 6.14

Check in with your client, asking, *"What is one word that describes how your body feels right now?"* If the client's experience is smooth, check in to see if she'd like to hold for another five breaths.

To release, roll over on to your right side, resting the head on the right arm. Pause here for a couple of breaths.

Bring the palm of the left hand directly in front of you, and press up to a comfortable seated position.

Check in with your client, asking, *"What is one word that describes how your body feels right now?"*

While there are other variations of Supported Fish that may lead to an even deeper release, remember that we are ultimately working on building energy here. Allowing release opens up space for building energy, hence our including it, but it is not the main purpose. After practicing a pose that allows release, make sure that you ground your client again via a couple of the grounding poses and/or breaths. Staff is a helpful *asana* to practice here, as the client is already in a seated position.

If the client is reporting feeling energized through these practices, and you are a psychotherapist, then you can work from here with other modalities you may typically use. If you are a yoga therapist, then now you can add practices that may be even more energizing, such as Revolved Triangle, Revolved Side Angle, or sun salutations. But remember not to ram the accelerator.

Regardless of where your client is, remember to start each session with a couple of grounding practices, and end with one grounding practice. And if you are a client who has been practicing some of this yourself and are feeling that your energy remains contained throughout, then you may now be in a place to explore a more general population vigorous yoga experience, and see if it fits your needs.

Vignette

Maria, a 62-year-old female, came to my office with symptoms of severe depression. She was having a hard time getting out of bed each morning, was not motivated to work (she was self-employed), was eating compulsively at night, and was crying frequently. Maria had experienced depression at many points in her life. Whereas she had been suicidal in the past, she denied suicidal ideation now. After I had worked with Maria on grounding for a couple of months, she began to focus on her work, and maintained a more regular schedule. She still complained of being low in energy and prone to lethargy and sadness.

Having introduced Maria to tratak *with the words "I am present" (see Chapter 5) previously, I now shifted gears into a visualization. "Think of one feeling that you would like to experience more in your life," I prompted. "What might that be?"*

"Love," she replied.

"Now, as you breathe in through the nose, imagine yourself filling with love," I guided. "As you breathe out through the nose, notice your body. Again, breathe in, imagine yourself filling with love."

As I guided, my eyes were on Maria, and I saw her squirm. "This is stupid," she said, "It's not going to work."

"What can we add so that it's more likely to be helpful?" I asked.

"I don't know," she responded despondently. "Give me a new brain. That might help."

"How about we go ahead and practice the breath for a few rounds," I suggested, "And then we'll check in at the end and see how we might adapt it in a way that's more helpful for you?"

"Okay," she responded grudgingly.

We began the visualization: "As you breathe in through the nose, imagine filling yourself with love. As you breathe out through the nose, notice your body."

Maria interrupted me. "It should be, as you breathe in, notice the love you have for yourself. Then, as you breathe out, notice your body."

I picked up the new phrasing with the next cycle: "As you breathe in, notice the love you have for yourself. As you breathe out, notice your body."

This was definitely an exercise in non-attachment for me as the therapist. From the start of our work together, Maria had voiced some resistance – often phrased along the lines of "How will this help me?" – to which I always responded, "Let's try it and see" – but this was the first time that she had expressed direct doubts (*"It's not going to work"*). Part of my challenge in meeting her in the moment was to meet the doubt rather than try to minimize it (via words such as "Of course it'll work") or take on a tone of authority (through a statement like "You're saying that because you're afraid").

Instead of being attached to what I was offering, I involved Maria in finding a way to make the practice work for her. I directly incorporated her concern that it would not be effective, and invited her to find a solution. Instead of saying, "Let's see if it works, and then if it doesn't we can change it," I suggested, *"What can we add so that it's more likely to be helpful?"* and *"we'll check in at the end and see how we might adapt it in a way that's more helpful for you?"* Notice that when Maria came up with an alternative, its words were actually far more definitive than mine had been.

Note also that the first sign of Maria's resistance was non-verbal: she squirmed. If I had not been attentive, I might not have seen that. I notice that when I lead yoga therapists in particular in these practices, they at times yearn so much to feel the effects of the experience themselves that they close their eyes as they're guiding. Your eyes as the therapist *must* always be open, both literally and figuratively. If my eyes had been closed, I would not even have been really present for Maria's verbal interruption, as it might have taken me a moment to come out of my "zone" to meet her.

References

Broad, W. J. (2012). *The science of yoga: The risks and rewards.* New York, NY: Simon & Shuster.

Telles, S., Nagathna, R., & Nagendra, H. R. (1996). Physiological measures of right nostril breathing. *Journal of Alternative and Complementary Medicine, 2*(4), 479–484. doi: 10.1089/acm.1996.2.479

Telles, S., Raghuraj, P., Maharana, S., & Nagendra, H. R. (2007). Immediate effect of three yoga breathing techniques on performance on a letter-cancellation task. *Perceptual and Motor Skills, 104*(3), 1289–1296. doi: 10.2466/pms.104.4.1289-1296

Weintraub, A. (2004) *Yoga for depression: A compassionate guide to relieve suffering through yoga.* New York, NY: Harmony Books.

7   Calming and Soothing

If we are working with a client who is experiencing agitation (*kṣipta*), then after we have worked with grounding, it may be time for us to move to building energy via a *langhana* practice. In the same way that we determined readiness to shift to a *brahmana* practice, we know when the client is ready to move to a *langhana* one: when they are consistently reporting feeling stable and grounded via the practice of the poses and breathwork described in Chapter 5. To return to the quote from Chapter 6: "A good yoga practice … involved poses that cycled through the accelerator and the brake" (Broad, 2012, p. 95). With *langhana*, we are working on the brake.

Just as with applying the accelerator, operating the brake is something that we cannot do thoughtlessly. If the car is moving rapidly and we employ the brakes suddenly and forcefully, it will just come to a screeching halt in the middle of the road, risking a collision. Under certain conditions, it may even skid and crash. So, once more, we are working mindfully, applying the brake gently and gradually.

Who Benefits from a *Langhana* Practice?

A *langhana* practice addresses *kṣipta*, or agitation, and therefore it is optimal for anxiety disorders such as generalized anxiety disorder, panic disorder, social anxiety disorder, and phobias. It is also appropriate for obsessive-compulsive disorder (OCD) and related disorders such as body dysmorphic disorder and trichotillomania, where a person turns to control in an attempt to manage anxiety. We will also discuss using *langhana* practices for attention deficit hyperactivity disorder (ADHD). As we mentioned in the previous chapters, a *langhana* practice is not appropriate when anxiety exists alongside a *mudha*-related condition such as depression or the potential depression present in bipolar disorders.

What Does a *Langhana* Practice Entail?

A *langhana* practice is about calming, which typically correlates with cooling. This can happen via:

- Poses that involve a forward bend of some sort.
- Breaths where the exhale is through the nose, and longer than the inhale.
- Combing holding a pose with a slower breath pattern, especially on the exhale.
- Cues to relax the muscles, including the jaw muscles.
- Visualizations and other suggestions of release, whether physical (releasing tension in the muscles) or metaphorical.
- A closed- or open-eyed practice. Whereas we were concerned to keep the eyes open with grounding and *brahmana* practices, closing the eyes can calm an agitated mind and allow the client to lengthen the breath further.
- A practice at any time of day. In the morning, a *langhana* practice allows a person to start the day from a calmer place. In the evening, it allows smoother sleep. Ideally, you would meet with your client closer to morning time, and give her a takeaway for both the morning and the evening.

Beginning a *Langhana* Practice

Just as with a *brahmana* practice, as you shift to a *langhana* practice, you still have grounding in mind. However, if your client arrives too agitated to work with grounding poses, the following warm-ups allow him to lean briefly into the energy of the agitation before working to contain it and ground. As we did with both grounding and *brahmana* poses, remember to introduce practices gradually. Allow time between one session and the next to assess the long-term impact on your client before adding hold time within a pose/breath or repetitions of poses/breaths. And as with *brahmana*, always end with a grounding practice.

Once more, one of the most important things to keep in mind is where we meet the client. As in the analogy in the previous section, if the client is highly agitated and I begin with a practice that is too slow, it is as if I were abruptly slamming on the brakes, therefore increasing the potential of a skid or a collision. I want to meet the client where he is, and in this case start just a tiny step *below* his energy level. If his voice is fast and frantic, mine is just a fraction slower, and just slightly less animated. Rather than starting in stillness and silence, we will begin with movement and sound. Be deliberate with your choices. Starting standing is generally helpful, unless it does not work physically for your client.

The Go-To Practice

In Chapter 4, we discussed takeaways, mentioning that we would return to them in this and the next chapter. Takeaways are an especially significant part of a *langhana* practice. Performing something regularly in the morning and the evening can be very helpful; even more beneficial for the short term is giving your client a go-to practice to which he will turn in a moment of acute crisis. This can be at the first signs of a panic attack for someone experiencing panic disorder, at the moment of wanting to pull out hair for someone with trichotillomania or carry out a compulsion for someone with OCD, or right before a social situation for someone with social anxiety disorder.

As you are moving through practices with your client, both of you can keep your eyes open for one that can be used as a go-to. You want this to be the practice that gives the client the most "bang for her buck," that is, the maximum effect in the minimum amount of time. You also want it to be portable, so that she can practice it wherever she is. So, while sun salutations may be an excellent general takeaway for your client, it is challenging to do them in the moment when the first symptoms of a panic attack rear their heads in public. You may advise your client to start her day with sun salutations at home, but suggest that she turn to a certain breath in a moment of crisis.

The go-to practice should have a grounding element, in addition to the calming it might bring. Since your client will be practicing in a moment of crisis, when he is probably in *viksipta*, you want the practice to help him stabilize first. See the vignette at the end of the chapter about an experience when that was not the case.

Warm-Ups

These warm-ups can be tried out independently first to assess where the client needs to start, before progressing to use them before other practices. Be careful of stimulating the client too much by moving too vigorously. It can be easy to think that a more intense practice will help the client get some agitation out of her system, but remember that your goal here is to meet the client a little *below* where they are and gradually move them down. I have heard many stories of people whose agitation has been increased via a practice that was too stimulating.

Shaking Things Out

If the client arrives with a high level of agitation, you can spend a moment (and only a moment) shaking things out, before moving to a calming breath and your grounding practice.

Come to standing. If that is not accessible physically, come to a seated position on a chair.

Notice how your body feels, and begin to shake out your arms and legs. Go with the speed and movement that feels right for this moment. I'll let you know after 30 seconds have passed, so that we can begin to bring the movement to stillness. If you'd like to stop sooner, feel free to do that.

(After 30 seconds from start of movement) *Now that 30 seconds have passed, allow the movement eventually to come to stillness. You can slow it down gradually if you'd like, eventually coming to stillness. I will let you know when 30 more seconds have passed, and if you have not come into stillness yet, please do so then.*

(After 30 seconds from the start of the slow-down, if the client has not stopped the movement yet). *Now that these 30 seconds have passed, allow your body to come to stillness. Notice how your body feels. Notice your physical sensations. Notice your breath.*

Take a deep breath in through the nose, bringing the arms up, so that the palms meet overhead.

Exhale through the nose, bringing the arms back down. Repeat once.

Check in with your client, asking, *"What is one word that describes how your body feels right now?"*

Notice that in this sequence, you are allowing the client a chance to express the level of agitation with which she is coming in, after which you are guiding containment. After she has had a chance to slow down her body, you are offering her a calmer breath, an evolution that feels smoother than if you had started with the breath. Your client gets to check in with a word at the end of the sequence, so that you can see where it took her.

The 30-second windows are important. The time is long enough for the client to move as she wishes, and then slow down as she desires. You are not rushing her, but at the same time, you are placing a limit on leaning into the agitation. By guiding the client to slow down at her own pace, you are giving her the space to move with, and then gradually shift away from, her agitation. You may be tempted to have your client exceed the two 30-second windows in the hope of reaching some sort of "catharsis." However, contrary to older theories that propose that releasing emotions such as anger is helpful, more recent research (e.g., Bushman, 2002) suggests that leaning into anger actually increases it. The goal, rather, is integration.

Make sure that you are clear with your instructions, outlining them as I did earlier. When we do not know what will happen next, that raises our anxiety, whereas when we do, that helps to calm us. Your clear instructions about how long the client will spend and what she will do at each stage empower her, and enable her to move in ways that work for her. And remember not to label the movement. Do not say, "Here's something that will calm you down." Your client may hear that as you shutting down her agitation, as others in her life may have done, telling her to "chill out." She may also not feel calmer at the end, and you want to allow room for that.

Empty Coat Sleeves

This is another technique where the client gets to lean into his agitation, and then gradually slow down and therefore move away from it. In general, you want to do either this or the previous technique, not both. However, if you ask for the client's word after the previous movement and receive a response that indicates continued agitation, you can move on to this technique. If you receive a word that suggests calm, then do not – you will just be stirring things up again and then trying to calm them once more.

Stand with your feet hip-width apart.

Begin swinging your arms back and forth as if they are empty coat sleeves. Allow your shoulders to be relaxed. You can look up "empty coat sleeves yoga" on YouTube to get a sense of the motion.

For the next 20 seconds, you may speed up the movement if you wish, allowing it to become as fast as you would like in this moment. You may also slow it down if that feels more natural.

(After 20 seconds) *Now begin slowing the movement down gradually, taking your time to come to a complete stop.*

Once the client has stopped, continue: *Take a deep breath in through the nose, and a deep breath out through the nose.*

Check in with your client, asking, "*What is one word that describes how your body feels right now?*"

Note that you are guiding your client for a briefer time through this movement than you did through the previous one, and that the breath that comes after it does not include a movement. That is because the arm movements in this pose are more powerful, being non-habitual and involving momentum. Try the two techniques yourself, and notice the difference.

Other Energetic Movements

If your client is still reporting feeling agitated, you may now shift to energetic practices that gradually move towards calm. In our first two movements in this chapter (shaking things out and empty coat sleeves), we began with a faster movement, invited the client to speed it up, and then to slow it down. You can lead your client through any of the energizing warm-ups from the previous chapter (pulling *prana*, hip swings, or pushing into the wall) or even the universal warm-up from Chapter 5, following a similar pattern. While you would not invite your client to speed up movements with more physical mobility such as these, you would start by guiding him through one or two "full strength" variations, and then invite him to slow the movement down slightly each time.

Pulling Prana Variation

Stand with your feet hip-width apart, or if that doesn't work for your body, come into a comfortable, grounded seat.

Reach your arms up, while inhaling quickly through the nose.

Exhale through the mouth quickly, as you pull the arms down (see Figure 6.1). *Repeat once.*

Now we'll move through the same movement, but we'll allow the pull down to be a little slower and a little gentler.

Once more, we'll move through the same movement, and allow the movement to be a little slower and a little gentler than this previous time.

And one final time, we'll move through the same movement, and allow the movement to be even slower and gentler this time.

Now come into one sun breath, inhaling through the nose as you bring the palms together overhead, and exhaling through the nose as you bring them down to your heart center.

Check in with your client, asking, *"What is one word that describes how your body feels right now?"*

The same approach can be used with hip swings, pushing the wall, or the universal warm-up.

Lion Pose

Lion pose brings in some humor, if that is accessible to your client in that moment, while at the same time allowing a slight calming. I always like to explain that it provides a mechanism via which to release tension, so that a client does not think I am taking his concerns lightly and suggesting a childish pose. And if there is any chance that your client might think that, then avoid that pose and go to others.

Start standing or seated. Inhale through the nose, and as you exhale stick out your tongue with a loud "aaagh" sound, allowing your eyes to look up towards the point between your eye brows. Repeat three times, allowing each sound to be a little less intense and a little quieter.

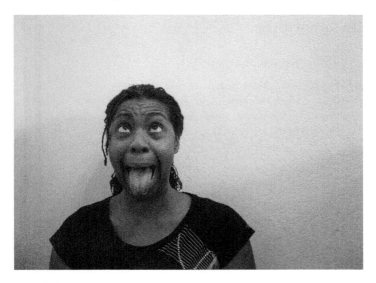

Figure 7.1

Check in with your client, asking, *"What is one word that describes how your body feels right now?"*

Sun Salutations

Another option is to guide your client through sun salutations, if you are comfortable doing so. Leading your client through a few rounds of sun salutations that you gradually slow down can be helpful to begin to work with *ksipta*. The universal warm-up sequence serves well to prepare the body for those movements.

If you are a yoga instructor and know that the traditional sun salutations that you typically lead would work for your client, feel free to guide him in those. You may go through a maximum of five sun salutations, allowing each to be a little slower than the previous one. One way to slow them down is to guide two or three as you typically would, and then with each round add one hold of one of the poses. So, for example, maybe in the first round you add a five-breath hold of downward dog. The second round keep that hold, and also add a five-breath hold of *ardha uttanasana* (half forward fold). Avoid holds that require more physical strength, such as *chaturanga dandasana*/bottom of a push-up. This is for two reasons: 1) we are working towards calm, and these are not calming poses, and 2) holding poses that are generally more physically challenging often correlates with holding the breath, which increases anxiety.

If you are not a yoga instructor and/or your client is not a regular practitioner of sun salutations, here are two variations through which you may choose to lead her. You may mix and match the poses in each. One makes use of the wall, and one does not. Note that the variation that is best for your client is the one that allows him to be most in the body, not tied to accomplishment and the ego.

VARIATION 1: SUN SALUTATIONS USING THE WALL

Come to stand facing the wall. You can also sit in a chair.

Inhale the arms up. Exhale, hinge forward, bringing your hands to the wall at as straight a line from the shoulders as works for your body. Press the hands firmly into the wall.

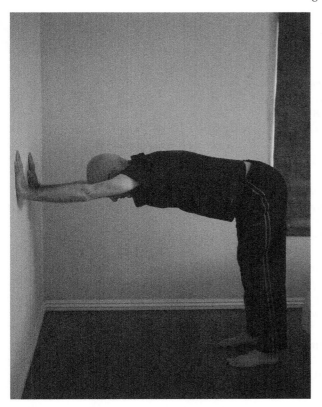

Figure 7.2

Inhale, bring the arms up a little bit up the wall.

Exhale, fold forward, walking the hands down the wall as far down towards the floor as works for you.

Inhale, bring the hands back to the wall (as in Figure 7.2 or its seated equivalent), *and press firmly.*

Exhale, keep the hands where they are, but release the firm press.

Inhale, walk the hands up the wall, and then slowly move them away from the wall, and up by your ears like in Mountain pose.

Exhale, bring the palms together at the heart center.

Check in with your client, asking, *"What is one word that describes how your body feels right now?"*

VARIATION 2: SUN SALUTATIONS USING THE FLOOR

Come to stand at the front of your yoga mat.

Inhale the arms up, hooking the thumbs together.

Exhale, release your torso forward, with the thumbs hooked together.

Inhale, bend the knees and bring the hands to or towards the floor.

Exhale, step the right foot back, coming into a lunge. You may use blocks if you wish (see Figure 6.8).

Inhale, step back to plank (top of a push-up) or all fours.

Exhale, bring the knees to the floor, and reach the buttocks back towards the heels.

Inhale, bring the chest forward, coming into Cobra or Cow pose (see Figures 6.12 and 5.5).

Exhale into downward-facing dog (see Figure 5.6).

Inhale, step the right foot forward, coming into a lunge. You may use blocks if you wish.

Exhale, step the left foot forward.

Inhale, hooking the thumbs together, bend into the knees, and raise the torso so that you're standing again.

Exhale, bring the palms together in front of the heart.

Check in with your client, asking, "*What is one word that describes how your body feels right now?*"

Note that these sun salutations eliminate movements that build energy, such as *chaturanga dandasana* (bottom of a push-up) and upward-facing dog (a pose that is similar to Cobra but with the knees off the floor, and that is typically practiced in place of the Cobra/Cow options given here). Rather, they balance calming poses with enough energizing ones that the calming is not too incongruous for the client at this point. For example, plank is maintained as an option, but instead of the heat-inducing *chaturanga* and upward dog, we have the less heating movements of bringing the knees to the floor and the buttocks towards the heels, and of Cobra/Cow, so that we are not increasing energy and, potentially, agitation. After all, in this context your goal is not to build your client's upper body strength, but to soothe and calm.

Building the Practice: *Asanas*

When your client's agitation shifts a little, you can move to poses that still engage the body, but calm the mind more.

Mountain with Slow Arm Release

Come into Mountain pose (see Chapter 5).

Hold the arms up by the ears for a few breaths. Then release the arms slowly, taking five long deep breaths to bring them all the way down by your sides. Notice sensations in your body as you bring the arms down.

Check in with your client, asking, "*What is one word that describes how your body feels right now?*"

Standing Poses Category 3 – Poses Emphasizing Release

Among the categories of poses we discussed in Chapter 5 were those emphasizing release, all of which involve a forward bend. This category includes Pyramid (*Parsvottanasana*), which we saw in the moon salutation (Figure 6.7), Forward Fold (*Uttanasana*), which we encountered in the sun salutations, and Wide-Legged Forward Bend (*Prasarita Padottanasana*). These are helpful to incorporate as we build a *langhana* practice, since they still ground the body via standing, but then allow the start of a calming practice. If you have a client with unmedicated high or low blood pressure, or someone who felt light-headed when you led her into the puppy stretch of the universal warm-up (Figure 5.2), you may wish to forgo this category of movements.

Wide-Legged Forward Bend

This is one of only two wide-legged poses that are included in this book. As mentioned previously, wide-legged poses can be triggering for clients with a history of sexual abuse or assault. However, when it comes to forward folds, it is easier physically to have a wider stance, and that stance from standing (versus seated or lying down) feels different in terms of safety for some (note the emphasis on "some").

If you are at this juncture, it means that you have worked with your client for a while, moving with her through grounding poses and other calming practices. Hopefully, the relationship between you is such that if you ask her about her comfort level doing a forward bend with a wider stance, she would feel safe answering you honestly. If it is not, or if she is doubtful, then guide her through the forward fold we encountered in the sun salutations instead, with the feet hip-width apart. With this, as with any other potentially sensitive practice, remember the words: if in doubt, leave it out.

Come to standing, and then step the feet wide. Place the hands on the hips, and begin to hinge forward. Bring the hands to blocks, the floor, or your legs. If you have unmedicated high or low blood pressure, you want to keep the back parallel to the floor, so that the head and neck are in line with the heart. Otherwise, let the torso fold forward, and let the crown of the head reach down towards the floor. You may rest the crown on a block if it is close enough to the floor.

To come out of the pose, bring your hands to your legs if they're not there already. Slowly walk your hands up the legs, till they arrive at the hips. Once they're at the hips, slowly raise the torso up. Step the feet together, and bring the palms together in front of your heart area.

Check in with your client, asking, *"What is one word that describes how your body feels right now?"*

Make sure that you guide your client to hold very briefly here at first (a couple of breaths), in case he might become light-headed. Once you know that the pose does not bring about any adverse physical effects, you can guide him to hold for up to five breaths.

Yoga Mudra *with Focus on Arm Release*

Come to a seated position on your heels. Feel free to place a block or blanket there to sit on, if you'd prefer. Interlace your fingers, or if that doesn't work for your shoulders, hold a strap.

Hinge forward, bringing your forehead to the floor. Or you may choose to bring it to a block, blanket, or pillow if you'd prefer.

Bring the arms as far from the back as works for you. Take a couple of breaths here. If your shoulders hurt when you do this and you have your hands clasped, come slowly back up to the starting position and try the movement with a strap instead.

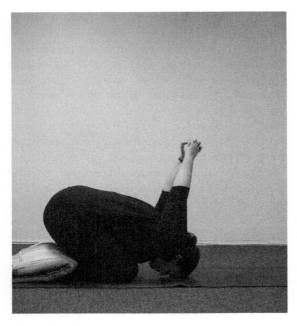

Figure 7.3

Keep the hands clasped or holding the strap, and come up. Only once your buttocks come to your heels, then unclasp your hands/release the strap, and allow your hands to float to your lap. Pause here for a couple of breaths.

Check in with your client, asking, *"What is one word that describes how your body feels right now?"*

Yoga mudra may be translated as "symbol of yoga." The pose is so named because the head is below the heart, signifying that the thinking mind is prioritized below the knowing heart. The symbolism of the pose is powerful, as is the sensation that may be felt at the time of the release of the hands. Make sure that the torso has returned completely to the upright starting position before unclasping the hands in order potentially to feel this effect, and be aware that the effect may be diminished by the use of a strap.

Head to Knee

Sit with both legs in front of you. Feel free to sit on a blanket, or to place a rolled blanket underneath your knees. Bend your left leg, placing the sole of the left foot against the right inner thigh. Bend forward, bringing your hands to either side of your leg, anywhere on your leg, or to hold a strap around your right foot. Hold for two breaths.

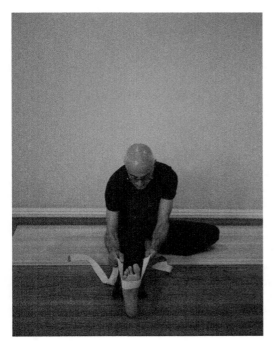

Figure 7.4

Slowly raise the torso, and switch sides. Bend your right leg, placing the sole of the right foot against the left inner thigh. Bend forward, bringing your hands to either side of your leg, anywhere on your leg, or to hold a strap around your right foot. Hold for two breaths, raise the torso, and come to a comfortable seated position.

Check in with your client, asking, *"What is one word that describes how your body feels right now?"*

As you guide the client through this pose and find that he maintains stability in the two-breath hold, feel free to continue adding gradually to the length of the hold, up to whatever amount of time may be comfortable for him. Note that, as opposed to a full straddle with the legs in a V-shape, the leg position in this pose may feel less open and therefore safer for a client with a history of sexual abuse or assault. Again, check with your client, and if in doubt, leave it out.

Beginning and Building the Practice: *Pranayama* and Meditation

There are changes that we can make to the length and type of breath to calm and soothe the body.

Left Nostril Breathing

As Telles, Nagathna, and Nagendra (1996) have demonstrated, inhaling and exhaling out of the left nostril is cooling and calming for the body. This is something that you may maintain for longer than we did for right nostril breathing, as there is not the same risk of hyperventilation if improperly executed. Always start and end with a few rounds through both nostrils, as we did in the previous chapter.

Sit in a position that is comfortable. Place your palms so that they are touching your lap. Keep your eyes open.

Inhale for a count of two, reaching the crown of the head towards the ceiling. Exhale for a count of two, relaxing the shoulders. Repeat twice.

Block your right nostril with the thumb of your right hand. Keep the left hand where it is. This is the opposite of what we did for right nostril breathing in Chapter 6.

Inhale through the left nostril for a count of two, reaching the crown of the head towards the ceiling. Exhale through the left nostril for a count of two, relaxing the shoulders. Repeat up to eight times.

Release your right hand back to your lap. Notice a word that describes how you feel in your body right now, and keep it in mind without speaking it out loud. Now inhale for a count of two through both nostrils, reaching the crown of the head towards the ceiling. Exhale for a count of two through both nostrils, relaxing the shoulders. Repeat twice.

Check in with your client, asking, *"What is one word that describes how your body feels right now? And what was the word that described how you felt right after breathing through the left nostril?"*

Exhale with Visualization

Another way to calm the body is by increasing the length of the exhale relative to the length of the inhale. We can again emphasize length by adding a visualization. In contrast to what we invited in Chapter 6 – what the client would like to bring in to her life – now we can ask her for something she would like to release from her life. I like to ask for that word before we begin the visualization to make sure it is not punitive (e.g., being fat, being a loser), and to give it power by being voiced.

Come into a comfortable seated position, with both hands on your lap.

Think of something that you would like to release from your life. Check in with your client, *"What might that be?"* Now, *inhale, filling your lungs with air, and as you exhale through the nose, imagine yourself releasing _____ (insert the word(s) here). As you inhale through the nose, fill your lungs with air. Again, breathe out, imagine yourself releasing _____. Now continue three more times at your own pace.*

Check in with your client, asking, *"What is one word that describes how your body feels right now?"*

Bhramari *(Bee Breath)*

As mentioned in Chapter 6, this breath can be energizing or calming, depending on the person practicing. Here, we will practice the traditional variation. You can look up *bhramari* on YouTube to get a sense of how it might sound.

Since your client's eyes and ears will be blocked, it is best to agree beforehand on a method to indicate that it is time to end the breath. Perhaps you will use a chime, if you have one, or set a soothing-sounding alarm on your phone.

Cover your eyes with the first two fingers, place the ring fingers under the nose, and the pinkies under the lip. Cover the ears with the thumbs. On an exhale, begin humming with the mouth closed. When you run out of breath, inhale and start again. Continue until your hear the "stop" signal.

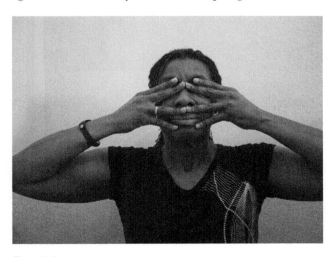

Figure 7.5

Allow your client to hum for about 30 seconds. End in the agreed-upon way. Check in with your client, asking, *"What is one word that describes how your body feels right now?"*

If *bhramari* turns out to be disquieting for your agitated client – if he reports tension or irritability, for instance – then, as with anything, simply repeat their word and move to the next practice.

Shitali/Sitkari

Both these breaths are atypical in that they involve an inhale through the mouth and an exhale through the nose. This is cooling, but also should not be practiced by the average person for too long, as inhaling through the mouth can be drying, and also reminiscent of hyperventilation.
Furl your tongue, protruding it a little beyond the lips. Inhale here.

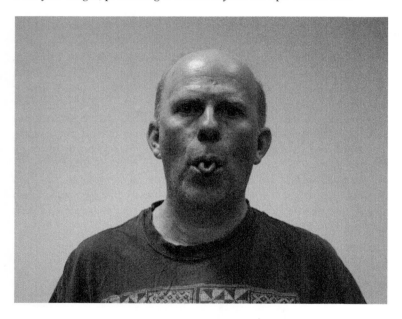

Figure 7.6

Close your mouth and exhale through the nose. Repeat twice.
Check in with your client, asking, *"What is one word that describes how your body feels right now?"*
If you are unable to furl your tongue, then you can try *sitkari* instead.
Place the tip of the tongue at the roof of your mouth. Allow the mouth to be opened just enough to allow the air to flow in. Inhale.
Close your mouth and exhale through the nose. Repeat twice.
Check in with your client, asking, *"What is one word that describes how your body feels right now?"*

Counting the Breath

Here, the client simply counts each breath until he arrives at ten, at which point he starts the count at "one" again. Allow the client to do this for about 30 seconds at first, and then you can lengthen the time.

Take an inhale. Take an exhale. This is one breath. Inhale again, and exhale again. Two. Inhale again, and exhale again. Three. Continue counting. When you get to ten, or lose count, just simply start at one again.

You may have remarked that this breath involves equal inhales and exhales, and so it has a grounding element. However, it is also typically more effective when completed with the eyes closed than with them open, making it more appropriate for this juncture in the practice.

Additional Points about a *Langhana* Practice for Certain Diagnoses

OCD

When it comes to OCD, it is helpful for your client's sense of safety to provide a relatively predictable sequence, and just make one change at a time. Introduce poses one at a time. Once you have a set that works, practice it in the same order, and make only one change at a time.

For example, you may begin with the universal warm-up from Chapter 5. The client should already be familiar with it from grounding work, and now you are planning to add one pose at a time for calming. Perhaps you first lead your client through the sequence rapidly, and then gradually slow it down. Then, at the end, you add a *yoga mudra*, and check in with your client about how that was for her body. Now you practice that sequence with that one change, until it is familiar for the client. Then, when it is time to make the next change, you make sure it is just one alteration again, whether it is an addition or a substitution.

ADHD

When working with ADHD, we need to meet the client with a practice that engages the energy of the body and the mind while helping build both focus and balance. From there, we can work on calming. The following practices are energetic physically, and also include a flow of movements that the client needs to track and that therefore helps with focus (as opposed to a hold, where the mind can wander more easily).

Hara Kumbhaka

Stand at the back of your space, arms by your side. Inhale through the nose. Exhale with a "ha" through the mouth, as you step the right foot forward, bending the right knee. Bring the arms up. You are in a modified Crescent pose. See Figure 6.10.

Inhale through the nose, stepping back. Exhale with a "ha" through the mouth, as you step the left foot forward, bending the left knee. Bring the arms up. You are in a modified Crescent pose.

Inhale through the nose, stepping back. Exhale with a "ha" through the mouth, stepping to your right, feet out, arms in cactus. You are in a modified Goddess pose. See Figure 6.5.

Inhale through the nose, stepping back.

Exhale with a "ha" through the mouth, stepping to your left, feet out, arms in cactus. You are in a modified Goddess pose.

Inhale through the nose, stepping back. Interlace the fingers and reach up.

Exhale through the nose, bringing the clasped hands in front of the belly button.

Inhale through the nose, stepping back. Interlace the fingers and reach up.

Exhale through the nose, bringing the clasped hands down in front of the belly button.

Check in with your client, asking, *"What is one word that describes how your body feels right now?"*

Based on the client's response, potentially repeat the entire sequence. Gradually add repetitions if appropriate for the client's physical and emotional containment. If you notice that your client's energy is contained and his focus is maintained, you may now shift to calming practices.

Tibetan Rites

Rather than the static hold typical of *asana* practice, the Five Tibetan Rites are a system of repetitions of five *pairs* of movements. The system involves doing each of the pairs once, then doing each of them twice, then three times, continuing in this manner until each pair is practiced 21 times. This would obviously be a time-consuming practice, so we are going to practice each of the movements once, twice, and three and four times. As the movements become more familiar and the body gains strength, the number of repetitions can be increased.

The first two rites are not for the amateur practitioner, as the first involves spinning in a circle and the second includes a movement that puts pressure on the back. Our focus will therefore be on the third, fourth, and fifth rites. They are presented here with a slight change from the traditional variations, in order to be physically gentler and energetically more controlled.

Tibetan Rite #3

Come to a kneeling position, leaning forward, chin tucked in to the chest. To help with stabilization, bring the arms forward.

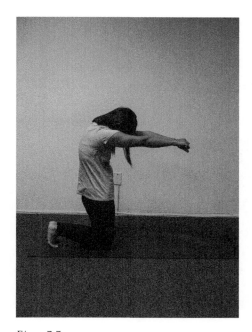

Figure 7.7

Inhale, bring the arms back, straightening the spine.

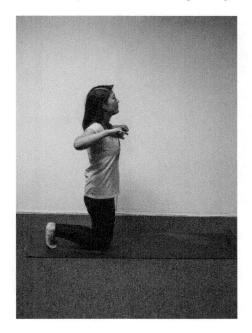

Figure 7.8

Exhale, return to the original position. Repeat twice more.

Tibetan Rite #4

Come to a seated position with the feet on the floor. Place the hands slightly behind you. Inhale here.

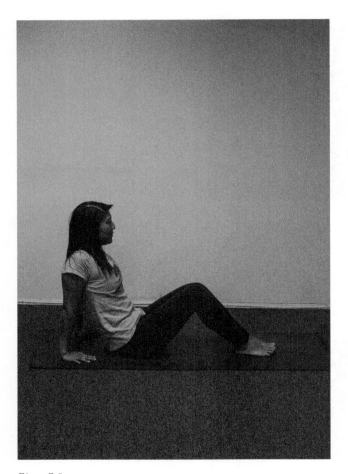

Figure 7.9

Exhale, and lift the buttocks off the floor, looking up at the ceiling. If this doesn't work for your body, then bring the shoulders back and down, accentuating the backbend of the spine, and allow the head to look up at the ceiling.

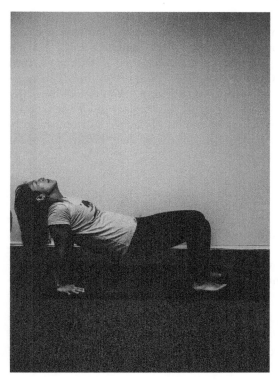

Figure 7.10

Inhale, return to the original position. Repeat twice more.

Tibetan Rite #5

Come to all fours. Inhale here.
   On an exhale, come to downward-facing dog (Figure 5.6).
   Inhale to upward dog (if your client is a seasoned yogi and you are a yoga teacher), *keeping your toes tucked under, and letting the transition be smooth.* (If your client is not a seasoned yogi and you are not a yoga teacher), *inhale to Cow pose* (Figure 5.5).
   Exhale to downward-facing dog. Repeat twice more.
   Check in with your client, asking, *"What is one word that describes how your body feels right now?"*

The traditional variations of these poses involve more back bending than we are incorporating here. As we are turning to them during a calming practice, we are limiting that movement so that we do not raise energy. Once your client has practiced each rite three times and had no adverse reports during the week, then you can practice everything three times, and then four times, adding in this manner.

If your client is a seasoned yogi, you are a yoga teacher, and you guide him through Rite #5 with the upward dog/downward dog pair, notice if the transition from one pose to the other is jerky and/or bouncy, putting pressure on the wrists in particular. If you do indeed remark that, then shift to the variation with Cow, as your client could get injured. Again, do not comment on the quality of the outward form, "You're looking jerky here, so we'll transition to Cow," but rather, just simply guide the practice and create the space for your client to notice, "Now we will transition to inhaling to Cow pose, and exhaling to downward dog. Notice how your body feels."

Balance Poses: Tree

This is the only time in this book that we will specifically turn to a balance pose, which can lead to a holding of the breath and a focus on achievement, both of which can result in anxiety. Balance poses can be helpful for building focus for clients with ADHD symptoms, however, as long as we select one that has different options for adaptability. Tree pose is one such example.

Stand with your feet together, hands on your hips. Then shift your weight to the left foot, picking up the right. Allow your gaze to settle on a point in front of you. This will be your focus point throughout the pose. Place the right foot on the ankle. If it's available, raise the foot further to the calf or the inner thigh.

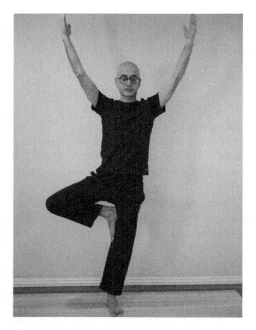

Figure 7.11

Bring the hands in front of the heart center. If you wish, bring them up from there and allow them to open. Hold here for three breaths, keeping your gaze on that same focal point.

If you lifted your hands away from the heart center, bring them back. Lower the hands from the heart center to the sides of the body. Slowly lower the right foot to the floor. Notice how your body feels.

Repeat the sequence on the other side. Check in with your client, asking, *"What is one word that describes how your body feels right now?"*

Insomnia

Insomnia may be caused by a number of things, and ultimately, when its cause is anxiety, decreasing the anxiety will improve it. Nonetheless, here are two sleep practices that you can offer your client to try at home. One is for stomach sleepers, and the other is for back sleepers. Note that the one for back sleepers may not feel safe for someone who is a survivor of sexual assault, as the legs are spread wide here. You can try out the poses in session, but do not leave your client in the pose to fall asleep. They need to sleep at night at home, not during the day in session!

Half frog (Svaroopa *Style*)

Come to a position lying on your stomach. Bend your right knee out to the right side, and if you like, place a folded blanket underneath the right inner thigh. Move the right knee and the right arm until the wrist and knee are touching. The left arm is down by your side, palm up. Bring your left cheek to the floor, so that your head is turned towards the bent knee.

Take long, deep breaths here. You may switch to the other side whenever you like. If you fall asleep here, then simply switch to the other side when you wake up.

Reclined Bound Angle

Place a rolled blanket or pillow just under the bottom tips of the shoulder blades. Lie back on it. Bring the soles of the feet together, knees wide. You may prop the knees with pillows too. Rest the hands wherever is comfortable. Take long, deep breaths here.

If the client is reporting feeling calm throughout the *langhana* practices, if you are a psychotherapist, then you can work from here with other modalities you may typically use. If you are a yoga therapist, then now you can add practices that invite even more stillness, such as meditation. But remember not to slam on the brakes too abruptly.

Regardless of where your client is, remember to start each session with a few grounding practices, and end with one grounding practice. If you are a client who has been practicing some of this yourself and are feeling grounded throughout, then you may be in a place to explore a general population gentle yoga experience, and see if it would fit your needs.

Vignette

Tyler was a 19-year-old male with a history of recent panic attacks. One day as he was driving home, Tyler passed an accident with a fatality. The car involved was the same make and model as his car, and it looked as if the driver who had been killed had been around his age. At the time, Tyler had a fleeting thought that that could have been him, and then moved on with his day.

The next day, when Tyler got in his car, his heart started racing and he began to sweat. As he started to drive, he was unable to breathe smoothly, and he had to pull over and text his mother to come and give him a ride. Tyler's mother was worried that he might be having a heart attack and took him to urgent care, where he was told it was "just a panic attack." In the three weeks since that incident, Tyler had been unable to drive, and had noticed his symptoms at a chronic low-grade level throughout the day. At certain times, however, they intensified, and while that always happened when he was in a car, that was not the only time they occurred.

At first I worked with Tyler on grounding. I did the 54321 grounding exercise with him frequently, as he often came into session with his symptoms at a heightened level from having to ride in the car to get to my office. As time went on, his symptoms were mitigated, but he was still unable to drive. As he reported feeling stable throughout the grounding practices, it was now appropriate to move on to some calming ones.

I introduced the pulling prana *exercise to Tyler. Maintaining his seated position in his chair, he did the exercise, starting more rapidly at first and then gradually slowing it down. He reported feeling calm afterwards, and we discussed making it his go-to practice. Tyler was enthusiastic and excited about that.*

The next week Tyler returned, reporting that he had turned to the pulling prana *practice, and it had intensified his panic symptoms. I was, of course, concerned.*

"What did you do then?" I asked.

"I don't know. I just lay in my bed, hoping I wouldn't die."

"That sounds terrifying. Then what happened?"

"After a couple of hours, my breathing started slowing down."

"So for you in that moment, breathing more slowly was what helped."

"Yeah, I guess so."

"Now that we know that breathing more slowly was helpful, let's try a different breath. Are you willing to try left nostril breathing?"

We did, and that became Tyler's new go-to pose. At first he was reluctant to use it, but then did so, and found it helpful. A few weeks later, as he began to feel calmer in general, I asked him if he was willing to guide me step-by-step through how he had practiced pulling prana, *so that we could learn what in it did not work for him. I asked him to narrate his progression in it for me.*

"Well, I was sitting like this," began Tyler, sitting in a hunched position on the couch, "And then I brought my arms up and pulled down." He then began moving quickly through the breath.

Immediately, I could how I had neglected to highlight the grounding necessary at the start of the pose when Tyler and I had practiced it in session before. I hadn't directly guided Tyler to create a stable base by pressing his feet into the floor or straightening his spine. In effect, he was working towards an energetic shift away from the panic without being fully in the present moment. The result was his spinning out of control.

"Thank you," I said. "I can see what in that practice doesn't work for you. Now what would be something we've learned that you could do now that would be helpful?"

Tyler turned to left nostril breathing, and I saw him relax.

Notice how throughout this experience, Tyler is in the driver's seat (no pun intended). While I am providing an opening into noticing what works for him, he is the one who decides what might help him. After all, he is the one who has to do that throughout his life, day-to-day. When he experienced a panic attack after pulling *prana*, he chose to lie down on his bed, and eventually his breath slowed down. As Trauma Sensitive Yoga founder David Emerson highlights, one of the most powerful experiences for a client is connecting "choices explicitly to what can be done with the body right now" (Emerson, 2015, p. 66).

When I asked Tyler to tell me about his experience of pulling *prana*, I asked him to narrate it to me, not just show me. This was to create some distance between him and the emotional response it might bring. Rather than saying, "Show me what you did," I prompted, "Tell me what you did."

I am also not tracking the story of whose responsibility it is that Tyler was practicing pulling *prana* in the way he was. I could have apologized and said I should have given clearer instructions, but I chose not to follow that track, since it would have taken us out of his felt experience and into our heads. Since we had found other practices that worked for Tyler, there was no need for us to return to pulling *prana* with more grounding cues. I now knew where my instructions had been lacking, so that I could guide Tyler more appropriately in other poses, and guide others more clearly in that one.

References

Broad, W. J. (2012). *The science of yoga: The risks and rewards.* New York, NY: Simon & Shuster.

Bushman, B. (2002). Does venting anger feed or extinguish the flame? Catharsis, rumination, distraction, anger, and aggressive responding. *Personality and Social Psychology Bulletin, 28*(6), 724–731. doi: 10.1177/0146167202289002

Emerson, D. (2015). *Trauma-sensitive yoga in therapy: Bringing the body into treatment.* New York & London: W. W. Norton & Company.

Telles, S., Nagathna, R., & Nagendra, H. R. (1996). Physiological measures of right nostril breathing. *Journal of Alternative Complementary Medicine, 2*(4), 479–484. doi: 10.1089/acm.1996.2.479

8 Working with Addictions and Eating Disorders

Now that we have explored how to apply the Three-Pronged Model with emotional health imbalances, we will examine its application in one other context: addictions (including eating disorders). Almost one in ten Americans (approximately 23 million) is addicted to alcohol or other drugs. The majority of that number (over two thirds) abuse alcohol, followed by marijuana, opioid (narcotic) pain relievers, and cocaine. In a nationally representative survey of adolescents, 52.4% reported alcohol use before age 16, 43.6% reported marijuana use, and 29.3% reported cigarette use (Butzer, LoRusso, Shin, & Khalsa, 2017).

In Chapter 2, we mentioned that the term "dual diagnosis" refers to the co-occurrence of an emotional health diagnosis with an addiction. Of the approximately 65 million individuals in the U.S. with a mental health diagnosis, an estimated 8.9 million have dual diagnosis (American Psychiatric Association, 2013). Let us see how the Three-Pronged Model can inform our work with chemical and behavioral addictions, including eating disorders.

Addictions

Addictions fall into two main categories: chemical and behavioral, although chemical addictions also include a behavioral component. For example, addiction to cigarettes includes a chemical addiction to nicotine, but cigarette use can also provide a social connection among smokers. Chemical addiction includes abuse of:

- Alcohol
- Marijuana
- Illegal drugs
- Nicotine
- Prescription drugs
- Glue/Solvents/Inhalants
- Food

The Diagnostic and Statistical Manual of Mental Disorders (DSM-5) uses the term "substance use disorders" to describe chemical addictions. A substance use disorder implies that the individual continues to use a substance despite significant related problems. These problems may fit under the overall categories of impaired control, social impairment, risky use, and/or pharmacological criteria. Impaired control refers to taking larger amounts of the substance than originally intended, unsuccessful attempts at cutting down, spending a great deal of time obtaining and using the substance, and/or craving the substance. Social impairment may comprise failure to fulfill major role obligations at work/school or home, persistent social or interpersonal problems, and/or giving up important occupational or social activities because of substance use (for example, the person may withdraw from family activities or hobbies in order to use). Risky use is consumption in physically or legally hazardous contexts.

Finally, pharmacological criteria refer to the *physical* reliance on the substance. Two ways to assess that are through tolerance and withdrawal. Tolerance is the need to increase amounts of the substance used in order to arrive at the same result. For instance, a marijuana user may find he needs to smoke more in order to feel the same "chill" effect he experienced before with less. Withdrawal is the development of a substance-specific syndrome when substance use is halted or decreased. A sign of withdrawal is the need to keep taking the substance in order to avoid withdrawal symptoms that appear when the person stops. An example of that is drinking coffee in the morning to avoid the headache you might develop if you don't drink it.

I gave marijuana as one of the examples in the paragraph above because with its legalization in many U.S. states, there can at times be a glossing over of its effects as "all natural." While cannabis derivatives have health benefits, like any substance, uncontrolled marijuana use can be problematic. In 2015, the National Survey on Drug Use and Health reported that over 4 million people in the U.S. abused or were dependent on marijuana (Substance Abuse and Mental Health Services Administration, 2017), and Winters and Lee (2008) found that those who begin using the substance before the age of 18 are four to seven times more likely to develop marijuana use disorder than those starting in adulthood.

As opposed to chemical addiction, which involves a substance, behavioral addiction (also called process addiction) refers to engagement in a particular behavior repeatedly, even if the behavior causes harm. Sometimes people are under the impression that behavioral addiction is not as problematic a behavior as chemical addiction. However, if you have ever known someone who is truly addicted to gambling or video games, you will have seen that while obviously the overdose risk is not present in behavioral addiction, the draw and intensity of the addiction can be as strong.

The DSM-5 expanded the previous category of "Substance-related Disorders" to "Substance-related and Addictive Disorders" in order to allow for behavioral addictions. Currently, the only disorder under the subcategory of 'Non-substance-related disorders" is gambling disorder, but behavioral addictions may also include:

- Gambling
- Sex
- Internet
- Shopping
- Video games
- Plastic surgery
- Food (binge eating or withdrawal)

Recovery from addictions is challenging, and the National Institute on Drug Abuse (updated 2014) estimates the percentage of people who relapse after a period of recovery to be between 50% and 90%, depending on the type of use. Reasons for relapse include not being "bottomed out" – that is, the client entered recovery for the sake of family/friends or for legal reasons – an unaddressed mental health condition, unrealistic expectations of the challenges of recovery, not dealing with the reasons for addiction, and spending time with the same people as before and continuing the same behaviors or mindset as before.

Eating Disorders

As mentioned earlier, food compulsion is one type of addiction. Sugar has been demonstrated to have chemical addiction properties (Avena, Rada, & Hoebel, 2008), and disordered eating (both overeating and undereating) are examples of behavioral addiction. Disordered eating refers to a variety of atypical eating behaviors that, by themselves, do not warrant diagnosis of an eating disorder. If these behaviors combine in particular ways that fulfill certain diagnostic criteria, then we refer to them as eating disorders.

Disordered eating is especially prevalent among young adult women. Mitchell, Mazzeo, Rausch, and Cooke (2007) report the results of one study in which 79% of undergraduate women evidenced symptomatology of an eating disorder, another in which 61% of the sample reported some form of eating disturbance – including subclinical bulimia nervosa, chronic dieting, bingeing, or purging – and a third in which 13.3% of undergraduate women demonstrated moderate or severe binge eating. Studies examining a broader range of disordered eating behaviors (e.g., extreme dieting) found even higher rates of disturbance

Anorexia Nervosa

A review of nearly 50 years of research (Arcelus, Mitchell, Wales, & Nielsen, 2011) confirms that anorexia nervosa has the highest mortality rate of any psychiatric disorder. The central aspect of anorexia is low body weight, in the context of what is minimally expected for a person's age, sex, developmental trajectory, and physical health. Anorexia involves a persistent restriction of energy intake leading to that low weight, combined with either an intense fear of gaining weight or continued behavior that interferes with weight gain. There is a disturbance in the way one's body weight or shape is experienced, undue influence of body shape and weight on self-evaluation, and/or a persistent lack of recognition of the seriousness of the current low body weight. Until the writing of the DSM-5 in 2013, anorexia nervosa was described only as a women's illness, as one of its criteria was amenorrhea (absence of periods). With the removal of that criterion in the DSM-5, the diagnosis can now be applicable to anyone if the other criteria are met.

There are two types of anorexia: restricting and binge eating/purging. The former is what we typically think of as anorexia, whereas the latter is what we characteristically consider to be behavior related to bulimia. However, when that behavior results in a significantly low body weight, that leads to a diagnosis of anorexia.

Bulimia Nervosa

Bulimia nervosa involves recurrent episodes of binge eating, followed by some sort of compensatory behavior. An episode of binge eating is characterized by both of the following: 1) eating, in a discrete period of time (e.g., within any two-hour period), of an amount of food that is larger than most people would eat during a similar period of time and under similar circumstances; and 2) a sense of lack of control over eating during the episode (e.g., a feeling that one cannot stop eating or control what or how much one is eating). After the binge, there is recurrent compensatory behavior in order to prevent weight gain, in the form of self-induced vomiting, fasting, excessive exercise, or misuse of laxatives, diuretics, or other medications. The binge eating and inappropriate compensatory behaviors both occur, on average, at least once a week for three months.

Binge Eating Disorder

Binge Eating Disorder (BED) is a new diagnosis that first appeared in the DSM-5. An episode of binge eating is characterized in the same way for BED as it is for bulimia nervosa, by both of the following: 1) eating, in a discrete period of time (e.g., within any two-hour period), of an amount of food that is larger than most people would eat during a similar period of time and under similar circumstances; and 2) a sense of lack of control over eating during the episode (e.g., a feeling that one cannot stop eating or control what or how much one is eating).

However, in BED, binge eating is not associated with the recurrent use of compensatory behaviors as it is in bulimia nervosa. Rather, binge eating episodes are associated with three or more of the following: 1) eating much more rapidly than normal; 2) eating until feeling uncomfortably full; 3) eating large amounts of food when not feeling physically hungry; 4) eating alone because of feeling embarrassed by how much one is eating; 5) feeling disgusted with oneself, depressed, or very guilty afterward. To qualify for the diagnosis, binge eating should occur, on average, at least once a week for three months, and there should be marked distress regarding it.

When it comes to recovery, traditional eating disorder treatment programs also have a low success rate. Dropout rates at inpatient programs for anorexia are at approximately 40% (Roux et al., 2016), and among patients who remain, about half relapse. Some researchers and clinicians think the missing key to long-term recovery may be rebuilding body awareness, and it is estimated that yoga is now incorporated in over half of residential eating disorder treatment in the U.S. to fulfill that need (Frisch, Herzog, & Franko, 2006).

How Yoga Can Help

Research (Butzer et al., 2017) points to five key ways in which yoga may prevent or reduce substance use:

- Reduction of stress and/or tension, and its overt behavioral and underlying neuroendocrine components.
- Reduction of depression, anxiety, and other mood imbalances, and a resulting increase in psychological well-being.
- Induction of a peak experience or higher state of consciousness, effectively replacing the attraction of a substance-induced high.
- Improvement in self-awareness and self-regulation of psychological and psychophysiological states, leading to the ability to intervene and prevent destructive or maladaptive behavior before its onset.
- The establishment of improved self-esteem and a better philosophical relationship and understanding between the individual and his/her internal and external (social) worlds.

Discussions of eating disorders point to the relevance of these elements in that context too. Binge eating (and disordered eating in general) can be motivated by a desire to escape from self-awareness, distracting attention from emotional distress and related negative cognitions (Baer, Fischer, & Huss, 2005). Consistent yoga practice encourages a greater connection over time both with one's body and with one's food consumption (McIver, McGartland, & O'Halloran, 2009b), and may be an effective adjunct treatment for reducing not only symptoms of anxiety and depression, but also weight and shape concerns in eating disorder patients (Hall, Ofei-Tenkorang, Machan, & Gordon, 2016). For instance, founder of Monte Nido eating disorders center Carolyn Costin describes, "Through yoga,

I developed a new kind of respect for my body, improving it with patience rather than pushing, and encouragement rather than the 'no pain, no gain' attitude I had been functioning under for many years" (2016, p. 28).

Therefore, some of the psychosocial advantages of yoga practice that we saw in Chapter 3 – building a greater consciousness of and connection to self – are especially healing from addiction and eating disorders. Ultimately, yoga allows for interoception, or attention to the inner physiological condition of the body, building an awareness of internal regulation responses, such as hunger. However, paying attention to the internal can be overwhelming, as it may involve noticing strong emotions that the client has been trying to escape via the addiction or eating disorder, and this is where developing dual attention that takes into account exteroception and grounding is key.

Before Meeting Your Client

Working with addictions can be challenging, and before doing so, you want again to examine your intention. What are you hoping to gain? Are your expectations realistic? While many recover, relapse is a constant specter in this work. Are you willing to work with someone who is just beginning a path to recovery, or with an active addiction? How will you handle the vicissitudes of that experience? Will you experience a sense of failure when you find out that your client has engaged in the addiction? Or can you focus on the here and now of the yoga session, without getting caught up in the story and becoming mired in self-doubt or shaming the client?

Starting with the Client

Contract

When working with addictions and eating disorders, there are contract rules that I believe are imperative to establish:

- While my role is not to shame the client if he has engaged in the addiction *between* sessions, if the client has a chemical addiction, he must be sober *during* the session. There is no point in practicing in an altered state, as what we are assessing in session will not even be relevant when the client is no longer impaired. This is something I establish from the start, and if the client comes to session high, I ask her in a kind but firm manner to leave (via a safe mode of transportation) and set up another appointment at another time.
- We will not discuss the effect of yoga on body size, shape, or weight. This is obviously especially pertinent in the case of eating disorders,

but can be relevant with other addictions too (such as in the situation of the smoker who might be worried about gaining weight after quitting, for instance). I frame this portion of the contract in broad terms: "We will focus on the internal experience, not the external form." Phrasing it in this way presents it as a general tenet rather than a specific rule that the client may take to be targeted at her and in response to which she may become defensive. This is something again that I outline at the start of our time together, so that I can remind the client of this aspect of the contract as appropriate. It also serves as a reminder to me not to fall into the trap of reinforcing external form, making statements about how a pose looks on the outside, rather than focusing on the client's experience of it (for more on this challenge as related to eating disorders, see Dunn, 2016).

• The yoga therapy that the client is undertaking with me is *complementary* to some other program, whether inpatient addiction recovery, a 12-Step program, a Self-Management and Recovery Training (SMART) program, or a Yoga of 12-Step recovery program (known as Y12SR and focusing on group yoga and processing sessions). Shifting addictive behavior or disordered eating is challenging, and it cannot be expected to occur in one or two yoga-based sessions a week. The structure, consistency, and community support provided by the client's recovery program are invaluable.

After I outline these points, I ask the client if there are other elements he would like to include in the contract between us that would help in his journey towards healing.

Assessment

Once the client and I have agreed on the contract, I move on to assess the circumstances under which he is tempted to turn to the addiction. I do not get into the story of how the client first started the behavior, but rather, what might draw him to it in the here and now. I keep this portion of assessment brief; there is no need to become lured into the seduction of describing the addiction or mired in the shame of it.

Generally, people turn to addiction for one, but sometimes both, of the following reasons:

• A shift in interaction. Sometimes, a person turns to addictive behavior out of a sense of emptiness, yearning to feel more connection. That might mean that she uses with others, bonds with others online, or generally feels isolated and relies on the addiction to escape that feeling. At other times, a person resorts to a behavior to move away from others.

- A shift in energy. A person uses the substance/behavior to feel either more energized/excited, or calmer.

Find out from your client which of these two reasons is important to him, and whether there is another source of motivation for the behavior. Sometimes people will use one substance to achieve one effect, and then another to mitigate that effect. The first feeling is the one you are seeking – the second typically just tempers it. And do not assume that the energetic presentation of a behavior is an indication of what your client is hoping to gain. For example, I have worked with many clients who turn to loud, violent video games as a means of self-soothing. The violence is noisy and intense enough to have a chance at taking attention away from the internal chaos they are experiencing, yet it is still more predictable than that internal disarray and therefore ends up being calming.

As we do with everyone else, we will begin by grounding the client. If the client is yearning for connection, we will incorporate that into grounding, via visualization and breathwork. However, we will use the Three-Pronged Model a little differently from how we have used it in the past, although the rationale behind that application is still consistent with the model.

First, we will be trying to *match* the state towards which the client yearns. This may feel contrary to what we have been doing before, when we were balancing excess dullness or agitation, but in fact we are following the same template. For example, let us say that someone uses alcohol to calm himself as he experiences anxiety. This would be a case of dual diagnosis, where there is both an emotional health imbalance and a substance abuse issue. But both ends of the dual diagnosis lead to the same conclusion. This person is experiencing an imbalance of *ksipta*, and so would benefit from a *langhana* practice. At the same time, he is self-medicating with alcohol, trying to "chill out," and so we will match the energy state he is seeking (calm) with a *langhana* practice.

The second way that we will use the model differently is that rather than staying only with grounding until we are sure that the client is feeling consistently stable, we will focus on grounding, but also incorporate limited *brahmana* or *langhana* practices. This is a client who already attempts to shift his energy, and we want to meet that. As we highlighted from the work of Butzer et al. (2017) earlier, one of the reasons that yoga may prevent or reduce substance use is via the "induction of a peak experience or higher state of consciousness, effectively replacing the attraction of a substance-induced high" (p. 605). While, of course, highs of this nature can in and of themselves become addictive (De Michelis, 2005), at this stage, this is a preferable attachment to the one held previously by the client. Over time, we can guide this client towards more balance and stability.

54321 Assessment

We have used the 54321 technique for both assessment (Chapter 4) and grounding (Chapter 5) in the past. Here, we will use it for assessment again – after, as usual, explaining to the client why we are using it – but with a slight twist:

Look around the room. Say out loud:

- *5 things that you see*
- *4 things that you're touching, or are touching you*
- *3 things that you hear*
- *2 things that you smell*
- *1 feeling in your body*

For our last prompt, rather than asking for a taste in the mouth, we are asking for a feeling in the body. We are doing this for two reasons. The first is that we are staying away from taste, for the sake of clients with eating disorders. The second is that we're using the 54321 technique itself as a transition from exteroception to interoception, in order to allow the client to notice what is happening internally without having to linger too much on it. In this way, we have an opportunity to assess the client's interoception in a far briefer manner, so that it is not overpowering.

If your client turns to look inward and is either overwhelmed emotionally or shuts down, that is an indication to you that turning inward is a challenge. Needless to say, you would not tell the client that, but it would be something of which you would be mindful. Being in the present can be challenging for all of us, and especially for those who have a history of escaping it in some shape or form.

Beginning the Practice

Recovery programs typically underscore taking things one day at a time, which is another way of highlighting the present moment that we are emphasizing in yoga. Our main point of focus is building that internal physical awareness. Mindful yoga classes, researcher and yoga therapist Laura Douglass (2011) explains, are an opportunity for students to learn how to discriminate between "bodily sensations" and "thoughts."

In order to do that, we will start with a few additional tools that help the client to tune into physical sensations – rather than thoughts or even emotions – before turning to some of the practices we have used in the past for grounding. We are helping clients to attend to internal feelings over external form, to prioritize "how do I feel?" over "how do I look?" (cf. Daubenmier, 2005). Ultimately, the aim is to help them tolerate sitting with discomfort, rather than trying to distract themselves from it

Grounding Through Body Awareness

In the first session, there are four practices that I like to explore with clients. Two begin the journey of building body awareness. The other two provide resources to which clients can turn between sessions.

The Gradual Breath

The breath (*pranayama kosha*) is a far more neutral place to start building awareness for a person with a history of judging herself by the appearance of her body. As we guide the client to focus on the breath, we will resist the temptation to suggest placing the hands on the belly in order to feel it. Not only might that pull the client with a history of disordered eating down the rabbit hole of evaluating the size of her belly, but it favors noticing external movement over internal sensations. With all our clients, we are moving away from using cues about the outside of the body as a substitute for sensations inside the body.

Take a deep breath in, and out. Notice your breath. Notice its length, and its depth.

Now breathe to only one third of your capacity. Pause for a second, then breathe out. Allow your breath to flow in and out normally for a few rounds.

Now breathe to two thirds of your capacity. Pause for a second, then breathe out. Allow your breath to flow in and out normally for a few rounds.

Now breathe to your full capacity. Pause for a second, then breathe out. Allow your breath to flow in and out normally for a few rounds.

Check in with the client: "*What is one word that describes how your body feels right now?*"

If breath control in this manner leads to anxiety for your client, check in to see whether just breathing part-way (without specifying a third or two thirds) might feel more organic.

Physical Markers

Pause, and notice your body sensations.

Notice your heart rate. What do you notice?

Notice your body's temperature. What do you notice?

Notice your level of thirst. What do you notice?

In this second practice, we are not asking the client to notice hunger or muscle tension, but rather, are developing awareness of more neutral and subtle cues. If your client responds with a story rather than a report of a present-focused physical sensation (for example, "I've been thirsty all day. I had to rush in the morning and I forgot my water bottle ..."), then gently guide him to the present moment, "And what sensations do you notice now?"

The Reset Pose

Typically, after these two practices – which I will use as the start for future sessions – I will outline two hallmarks of the practice to the client. The first is the reset pose, to be practiced a certain number of times per day for grounding. The reset pose is not aiming for particular results (e.g., moving away from an addiction). It is simply to be consistently practiced, regardless of what else is going on, for continuity and stability. The number of times it should be practiced daily can be determined through dialog between you and your client, but three to five times is generally reasonable.

One pose I commonly use for this purpose is downward-facing dog, since it involves grounding through the hands and feet, while literally also providing a new perspective.

Come to your hands and knees. Make sure that the hands are directly below the shoulders, and the knees are directly below the hips. Spread the fingers wide, with the middle finger pointing straight forward.

Press into your fingers, tuck your toes under, and lift your knees off the floor (Figure 5.6). *Keep your knees bent.*

Inhale, and continue to feel your fingers pressing into the floor. Exhale, and reach your heels towards the floor any amount. Repeat this two more times.

Bring the knees back to the floor, and come to sitting.

Check in with your client, asking, *"What is one word that describes how your body feels right now?"*

You will notice that this time, we emphasized grounding in this pose even more than we have in the past. We want to remind the client that when he does the pose, he can really notice that contact between his hands and the floor.

There are a couple of additional elements that you can bring to the pose. The first is an affirmation that comes naturally to the client. You can ask the client, "What is a quality you hope to cultivate?" and make that the affirmation. The client can then repeat the affirmation in her mind in synch with the breath; for example, breathing in "I am" and breathing out "strong."

The second is an add-on that matches the effect that the client is yearning for via his addiction. For example, if the client hopes to increase energy, perhaps you can add bending and straightening alternate legs, or transitioning from downward dog to plank, depending on your client's strength and energy (remember, you want to match the energy, not overdo it).

So, you might cue,

As you hold downward dog, inhale and bend into your right knee, straightening your left leg. Exhale and bend into your left knee, straightening your right leg. Repeat two more times.

Or

Now, from downward dog, inhale and shift your weight forward into plank (top of a push-up). Exhale back to downward dog. Repeat two more times.

On the other hand, if the client hopes to calm himself, then you can guide him into Child's pose after downward dog. While we stayed away from doing Child's pose right after downward dog in the past when working with grounding, now we are aiming to match the client's desired energy level a little, and so if he turns to an addiction for calm, we will make that accessible here.

Bringing the knees back down to the floor, now reach the buttocks back towards the heels. Rest your forehead on the floor or on a block.

With any of these add-ons, you want to make sure to check in with your client, asking, *"What is one word that describes how your body feels right now?"* If downward dog does not work for your client, an alternate reset pose I often use here is pushing against the wall, as described in Chapter 6 (Figure 6.2).

Stand facing the wall. Take a few steps back, and place your hands on the wall. Spread your fingers wide.

Step your right foot forward, and inch your left foot back. Bring the heel of your left foot towards the floor as much as possible. Bend your right knee, and make sure the knee doesn't go past the ankle. Press into your hands. Hold for three breaths. As you inhale, press into your fingers. As you exhale, relax your shoulders. Repeat.

Step your right foot forward, and inch your left foot back. Bring the heel of your right foot towards the floor as much as possible. Bend your right knee, and make sure the knee doesn't go past the ankle. Inhale here. Exhale with a "ha" sound, pressing into your hands. Inhale, releasing the pressure in your hands but keeping them on the wall. Exhale with a "ha" and press into them. Repeat twice.

The Go-To Practice

We introduced the go-to practice in Chapter 7, where it served as an anchor during times of particularly acute anxiety and agitation. Here, we will use it when the urge for the addictive behavior becomes strong. I explain the concept at the outset, so that the client is on the lookout for something suitable as we practice together during our session. Again, it should be something with which the client connected, which is portable, and which is easy to remember and execute. Perhaps it is the gradual breath we just practiced; counting the breath in rounds of ten as we did in Chapter 7 is another possibility.

In subsequent sessions, we can ask the client whether he turned to the go-to practice during the week. If he has not, we will refrain from asking why, but instead, inquire whether he feels that a different go-to practice might be more helpful. In this way, it is the client who decides what works or does not work in a way that places the responsibility on him without shaming him. And again, note your own expectations. If the client turned to the go-to practice even once, that means he used it.

Building the Practice

Building Grounding Through Body Strength

Grounding poses that use body strength are especially empowering for those who turn away from their emotions towards distraction, and in particular for those with disordered eating who have judged their body to be deficient in some way. The poses that we used in Chapter 5 for grounding can be incorporated, with particular emphasis on body strength. These poses were:

- Mountain
- Standing squat
- Downward dog
- Warrior II

We would guide these poses as we did in Chapter 5, with an additional emphasis on solidity that still allows for multiplicity of experience. We might say, "Notice what in your body feels solid," or, "Notice your legs," "Notice your arms," or "Notice your core," and allow the client to connect with whatever physical sensations she may be experiencing.

Building Grounding Through Breath and Visualization

Focusing on an even breath is a useful way of helping the client gain balance. Among the breaths that we may practice here are:

- Sun breaths
- Alternate nostril breathing
- *Tratak*, with focus on a mantra such as "I am present" or a candle flame
- Counting the breath

If the client has indicated that she turns to her addiction for connection (e.g., she uses with others, bonds with others online, or generally feels isolated and turns to the addiction to escape that feeling), we may also incorporate a related visualization. As it would resonate more to use her words, we can ask how she would prefer to feel, and then adopt those words for a visualization. For example, we may guide a *pranayama* practice in which she focuses on the words, "I am one with all." We want to direct the client to keep her focus on the breath as she practices this, so that her mind does not slip to the story, particularly since that could lead her down a path of memories of times when she did *not* feel that she was one with all.

Brahmana *Practices*

When it comes to matching highs, we would be working with some of the practices that we incorporated previously at the start of a *langhana* practice or towards the midpoint of a *brahmana* practice. Particularly helpful practices include:

- Pulling *prana*
- Sun salutations
- *Hara kumbhaka*
- Tibetan rites
- Right nostril breathing
- *Bhramari*
- Crescent pose with arm variations (discussed in the section on moon salutations)

Note that these practices share three characteristics: they are movements with shifts versus holds of the body, the torso is typically straight during them, and they include an even length and exhale (even if the exhale is through the mouth, as in pulling *prana*).

These characteristics enable us to focus on building energy while containing emotion to a certain extent. Practices such as backbends or the breath of joy, which also build energy, may move about too much emotion to be helpful. If the emotion moved is too intense, the resulting overwhelm can push the client towards the comfort and numbing of his addiction. And if your client reports feeling tired after a *brahmana* practice, then return to grounding.

Langhana *Practices*

When it comes to matching calm, we will work with some of the practices that we incorporated previously either at the start of a *brahmana* practice or towards the midpoint of a *langhana* practice. Particularly helpful practices include:

- Moon salutations
- Mountain with slow arm release
- *Yoga mudra* with focus on arm release
- Forward fold
- Left nostril breathing
- *Bhramari*
- *Shitali/Sitkari*

When it comes to forward folds, we want to be aware especially here of poses where the legs are far apart. There is a strong correlation between trauma and addiction, and we do not want potentially to trigger the client. Even when we think we know the client has no history of sexual abuse or assault, it is always prudent to err on the side of caution, especially since there are plenty of other practices to which we can turn.

Finally, an important aspect to remember when working with addictions is your own practice of *ahimsa*. You are providing a complementary modality for your recovering client, and your client's journey – like any other journey – involves its own highs and lows. If you find out after a practice that your client was so agitated that he immediately turned to the addiction for numbing, remember that this is his coping strategy in general, and that he has turned to it hundreds of times before under circumstances that had nothing to do with you. The experience provides the two of you with information on his window of tolerance, and you can adjust your work accordingly. The most important offering that you bring to him is your non-attachment to outcome.

Vignette

David is a 50-year-old male who was referred to therapy by his physician. After he passed out at the gym and was taken to the hospital, it was discovered that David had fainted several times during or after a workout. After a thorough check-up that revealed nothing noteworthy, David's physician remarked on David's being a little overweight. "Yeah, I know," David responded, "I got close to 50 and I just started gaining weight. So I've been trying to exercise more, but no matter how much I exercise, I don't lose any weight. I guess I eat too much." David's physician thought that perhaps David was depressed, and sent him to therapy.

As I was doing my intake with David and asked him about creative outlets, he mentioned exercise. I discovered then that he exercised for four hours every day. When I asked him what his motivation was for doing that, he explained that the quantity he typically ate necessitated it. I found out that he ate very large amounts of food in short spans of time almost every evening, and that he felt he had no control over what he ate. His eating patterns fitted the criteria for binges, while his exercising was excessive and compensatory. He therefore qualified for a diagnosis of bulimia.

David exercised in order to feel powerful and strong. He was eager to start yoga, as he had heard it could build strength, and wanted to focus on poses that developed muscle and served as a bridge to burn calories. I explained to him that in therapeutic yoga we were building strength and power in body, mind, and spirit, but that we were going to do it gradually. Otherwise, it would be like constructing a building with no foundation: it was just going to crumble. David looked at me with some skepticism, but he also did not outwardly reject what I was suggesting.

I introduced Mountain pose, standing squat, and downward dog, explaining that these were poses that helped to build that foundation, and that at the same time worked with and built on his strength. After the asanas, we incorporated breaths with a strong exhale, such as pulling prana and the breath of joy. At first, David was eager to learn more poses, but over time he settled into the breaths, and we added bhramari, as well as a visualization where as he inhaled, he envisioned strength and power.

While bulimia, like anorexia, is typically associated with women, it is also diagnosed in one man for every ten women. Bulimia in men more typically uses exercise as the compensatory practice. One of the biggest challenges in working with David was to help him access his strength without yoga becoming one more medium via which to exercise excessively. I met him where he was by emphasizing physical strength, offering him practices that did so but that also highlighted grounding and solidity. I incorporated some breaths to offer a complementary focus point (that of *pranayama kosha*) to the physical (*annamaya kosha*) and mental (*manomaya kosha*) that were absorbing his attention. From the start, I acknowledged what he was yearning for via his addiction – strength and power – and paid attention to that, while at the same time positioning those needs within a more holistic framework.

Note that David's doctor suspected that he might be experiencing depression. The practices that I gave him to match what he wanted were strengthening/energizing ones that fitted within a *brahmana* practice. Therefore, assessing David's practice via the addiction lens or the emotional imbalance lens would have led us towards the same path.

References

American Psychiatric Association. (2013). *Diagnostic and statistical manual of mental disorders* (5th ed.). Washington, DC: American Psychiatric Publishing.

Arcelus, J., Mitchell, A. J., Wales, J., & Nielsen, S. (2011). Mortality rates in patients with anorexia nervosa and other eating disorders: A meta-analysis of 36 studies. *Archives of General Psychiatry, 68*(7), 724–731. doi: 10.1001/archgenpsychiatry.2011.74

Avena, N. M., Rada, P., & Hoebel, B. G. (2008). Evidence for sugar addiction: Behavioral and neurochemical effects of intermittent, excessive sugar intake. *Neuroscience & Biobehavioral Reviews, 32*(1), 20–39. doi: 10.1016/j.neubiorev.2007.04.019

Baer, R. A., Fischer, S., & Huss, D. B. (2005). Mindfulness-based cognitive therapy applied to binge eating: A case study. *Cognitive and Behavioral Practice, 12*(3), 351–358. https://doi.org/10.1016/S1077-7229(05)80057-4

Butzer, B., LoRusso, A., Shin, S. H., & Khalsa, S. B. (2017). Evaluation of yoga for preventing adolescent substance use risk factors in a middle school setting: A preliminary group-randomized controlled trial. *Journal of Youth and Adolescence, 46*(3), 603–632. doi: 10.1007/s10964-016-0513-3

Costin, C. (2016). Yoga: A healing journey, from personal to professional. In C. Costin & J. Kelly (Eds.), *Yoga and eating disorders: Ancient healing for modern illness* (pp. 3–12). London & New York: Routledge.

Daubenmier, J. (2005). The relationship of yoga, body awareness, and body responsiveness to self-objectification and disordered eating. *Psychology of Women Quarterly, 29*(2), 207–219. doi: 10.1111/j.1471-6402.2005.00183.x

De Michelis, E. (2005). *A history of modern yoga: Patanjali and Western esotericism.* New York, NY: Bloomsbury Academic.

Douglass, L. (2011). Thinking through the body: The conceptualization of yoga as therapy for individuals with eating disorders. *Eating Disorders, 19*(1), 83–96. doi: 10.1080/10640266.2011.533607

Dunn, L. (2016). The shadow side of yoga. In C. Costin & J. Kelly (Eds.), *Yoga and eating disorders: Ancient healing for modern illness* (pp. 130–141). London & New York: Routledge.

Frisch, M. J., Herzog, D. B., & Franko, D. L. (2006). Residential treatment for eating disorders. *International Journal of Eating Disorders, 39*(5), 434–442. doi:10.1002/eat.20255

Hall, A., Ofei-Tenkorang, N. A., Machan, J. T., & Gordon, C. M. (2016). Use of yoga in outpatient eating disorder treatment: A pilot study. *Journal of Eating Disorders, 4*, 38. doi: 10.1186/s40337-016-0130-2

McIver, S., McGartland, M., & O'Halloran, P. (2009). 'Overeating is not about the food': Women describe their experience of a yoga treatment program for binge eating. *Qualitative Health Research, 19*(9), 1234–1245. doi: 10.1177/1049732309343954

Mitchell, K. S., Mazzeo, S. E., Rausch, S. M., & Cooke, K. L. (2007). Innovative interventions for disordered eating: Evaluating dissonance-based and yoga interventions. *International Journal of Eating Disorders, 40*(2), 120–128. doi:10.1002/eat.20282

National Institute on Drug Abuse website (Updated 2014). Drugs, brains, and behavior: The science of addiction, treatment and recovery. Retrieved April 6, 2018 from www.drugabuse.gov/publications/drugs-brains-behavior-science-addiction/treatment-recovery

Roux, H., Ali, A., Lambert, S., Radon, L., Huas, C., Curt, F., ... the EVHAN Group. (2016). Predictive factors of dropout from inpatient treatment for anorexia nervosa. *BMC Psychiatry, 16,* 339. doi: 10.1186/s12888-016-1010-7

Substance Abuse and Mental Health Services Administration (2017) Results from the 2015 National Survey on Drug Use and Health: Detailed Tables, SAMHSA, CBHSQ. Retrieved April 6, 2018 from www.samhsa.gov/data/sites/default/files/NSDUH-DetTabs-2015/NSDUH-DetTabs-2015/NSDUH-DetTabs-2015.htm

Winters, K. C., & Lee, C.-Y.S. (2008). Likelihood of developing an alcohol and cannabis use disorder during youth: Association with recent use and age. *Drug Alcohol Dependence, 92*(1–3), 239–247. doi:10.1016/j.drugalcdep.2007.08.005

Conclusion

Almost 20 years ago, mindfulness researcher Diane Reibel and her colleagues drew attention to the "high prevalence of psychological distress" in our society. "As the average age of our population increases and chronic illness rates expand," they urged, "it is imperative to develop and implement low-cost, effective, therapeutic interventions that help alleviate suffering and improve patient functionality" (Reibel, Greeson, Brainard, & Rosenzwig, 2001, p. 183). This imperative is even more needed now, as reports of emotional imbalance continue to rise: rates of depression in the United States, for example, increased from 6.6% in 2005 to 7.3% in 2015 (Weinberger et al., 2017).

The need for novel ways of working towards emotional well-being is clearly critical, and that includes learning to maintain emotional well-being, not just managing crisis. We are desperately in need of the preventive emotional health maintenance mentioned by Sat Bir Khalsa in Chapter 2. But instead, as Jon Kabat-Zinn describes, our society "persists in devaluating the present moment in favor of perpetual distraction, self-absorption, and addiction to a feeling of 'progress'" (2003, p. 148). We turn away from that present moment again and again, yearning for relief somewhere outside of ourselves. Yet it is in that moment and our internal self-awareness that the relief lies.

Especially during times of emotional difficulty, the overarching (and often overwhelming) response is experienced in the body. The angry person's breathing becomes more shallow, her face reddens, and her entire body tenses. The depressed individual's shoulders slump forward, his chest hollows, and his voice is barely audible. The person flooded by trauma becomes immobile and frozen, perhaps even unable to speak. In all these cases, it is their bodies, not their words, that tell their stories most expressively. And, therefore, it is through their bodies, not their words, that they can gently guide themselves to a place of greater stability and balance.

The yogic approach to treatment differs radically from current standards of care. Instead of a focus on symptom reduction through addressing negative thought patterns, troubling memories, or feared stimuli, yoga uses the body and breath to build awareness. As the client balances the exteroception towards his surroundings and the interoception towards his physical sensations and cues, he gains empowerment through that attunement. This approach differs from the typical medical model, which compartmentalizes healing and externalizes it to outside expertise rather than internal knowing. The spread of this educational model of healing is still in its infancy, and therefore, in your willingness to be part of it, you are on the cutting edge of a movement. Regardless of how much the practice of yoga has proliferated in the last two decades, its use therapeutically in this manner is still a relatively underexplored frontier.

If you are a therapist, as you adjust to working in this way, the most important thing to remember is to meet your client where she is, and progress according to the cues her body gives you, not those your ego or her ego may provide. Remember that your practice of non-attachment to the outcome of each practice models for her a flexibility that we do not tend to encounter in our day-to-day lives, especially as goal-oriented Americans. Do not be afraid of repeating practices – familiarity breeds comfort.

Yoga therapists, instructors, and practitioners are often eager to jump into deeper practices that they believe will create more rapid shifts. Remember that just as a building needs well-constructed infrastructure, so do we as human beings. Every client needs first to start with grounding work, and only transition gradually from that to energizing or calming practices once grounding has been clearly established. Over-engaging the body weakens our relationship to it. As yoga teacher, health counselor, and former Olympic athlete Jamie Silverstein powerfully highlights,

> Early on in my yoga practice, a teacher encouraged me to take a break from the physical movement so that I could listen to the hum of my body; not my mind, my body. This was a pivotal moment in my relationship to myself: there was something within me to hear.
>
> (Silverstein, 2016, p. 248)

As you encourage your client to listen to her inner wisdom, remember to listen to yours. Consult with more experienced practitioners as much as you need. Give your work your full attention at all levels and with all your *koshas* (body, breath, mind, wisdom, and maybe even bliss) when you are in session, and then let it go once you are out of session. Researching information and preparing protocols for your client outside of session is one thing, but being pulled into either self-praise about how well you guided or self-doubt about how poorly you did is the work of ego and attachment. It does not serve you or your client.

At any point during your session, if you are unsure of what to do, return to the two central premises of this work: grounding and meeting the client where she is. Remember that grounding helps both you and your client. Check in frequently. If you feel that your frequent check-ins or your pace is troubling your client, have a frank conversation with him about it. Explain your purpose behind it, and ask him what he would prefer, rather than ramming the accelerator or the brake based on assumptions. And if you are unsure about the suitability of a practice, err on the side of caution and omit it. If in doubt, leave it out.

If you are anticipating using this work for yourself, I am humbled that you have considered it as part of your healing journey, and hope that it serves you. If you are a practitioner – whether a psychotherapist or a yoga therapist – my hope is that you have benefited or will benefit from the central paradigm and framework in this book, and that you will also augment it and make the practices within it your own. My hope in providing a framework, not just a list of poses and breaths, is that the practices may serve as examples rather than mandates. One of the most exciting aspects for me as I train therapists in this work is seeing them personalize and enrich it.

There is much future work to be done in the realm of therapeutic yoga for emotional health. There is highly promising potential for therapeutic yoga to interface with other modalities such as eye movement desensitization and reprocessing (EMDR) therapy that focus on single-incident trauma, complex trauma, and resulting imbalances such as depression, anxiety, and trauma-related disorders (cf. Haas, 2016). Evidence-based research and outcome-based therapy with yoga for emotional health have grown exponentially in the last decade, and I look forward to the continuation of that evolution. I firmly believe that yoga holds the key to emotional healing, and am honored to make a small contribution in that direction. Thank you for having joined me on that journey.

References

Haas, L. (2016). Yoga for emotions: Tools for healing from eating disorder behaviors. In C. Costin & J. Kelly (Eds.), *Yoga and eating disorders: Ancient healing for modern illness* (pp. 176–193). London & New York: Routledge.

Kabat-Zinn, J. (2003). Mindfulness-based interventions in context: Past, present, and future. *Clinical Psychology: Science and Practice, 10*(2), 144–156. doi: 10.1093/clipsy.bpg016

Reibel, D., Greeson, J., Brainard, G., & Rosenzwig, S. (2001). Mindfulness-based stress reduction and health-related quality of life in a heterogeneous patient population. *General Hospital Psychiatry, 23*(4),183–192. doi:10.1016/S0163-8343(01)00149-9

Silverstein, J. (2016). Athletes, yoga, and eating disorders. In C. Costin & J. Kelly (Eds.), *Yoga and eating disorders: Ancient healing for modern illness* (pp. 237–249). London & New York: Routledge.

Weinberger, A. H., Gbedemah, M., Martinez, A. M., Nash, D., Galea, S., & Goodwin, R. D. (2017). Trends in depression prevalence in the USA from 2005 to 2015: Widening disparities in vulnerable groups. *Psychological Medicine, 12,* 1–10. doi: 10.1017/S0033291717002781

Index

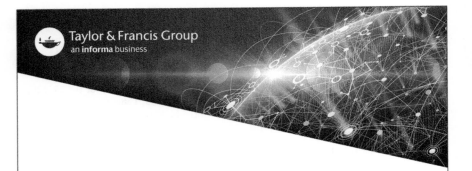